Resuscitation at Birth

Newborn Life Support

Third Edition

ISBN – 978-1-903812-25-9

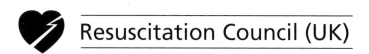

Resuscitation Council (UK)

Contents

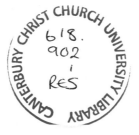

The Newborn Life Support sub-committee

In 1998 the Resuscitation Council (UK) brought together representatives of a number of professional bodies interested in resuscitation at birth to develop a standard training course for the United Kingdom. Pilot courses run in 1999 allowed the development of a course which has received support from all the appropriate parent bodies. The first edition of this manual, written by the original working party, accompanied the Newborn Life Support course which was launched in 2001. The publication of an updated consensus document by the International Liaison Committee on Resuscitation (ILCOR) in October 2010 provided the stimulus for updating this manual.[142, 209]

The Resuscitation Council (UK) Newborn Life Support sub-committee 2010:

Jonathan Wyllie	(Chairman) Neonatologist, James Cook University Hospital, Middlesbrough
Sean Ainsworth	Neonatologist, Forth Park Hospital, Kirkcaldy
Alison Bedford Russell	Neonatologist, The Women's Hospital, Birmingham
Andy Coleman	Senior educational advisor
Rowan Davies	NLS course coordinator, Resuscitation Council (UK)
Mervi Jokinen	Midwife, RCM Practice and Standards Development Advisor
John Madar	Neonatologist, Derriford Hospital, Plymouth
Stephanie Michaelides	Senior lecturer in midwifery and neonatal care, University of Middlesex
Sarah Mitchell	Director, Resuscitation Council (UK)
Niall Pearcey	Resuscitation officer, Norfolk & Norwich University Hospital
Sam Richmond	Neonatologist, Sunderland Royal Hospital
Vivienne van Someren	Paediatrician, Royal Free Hospital, London
Rob Tinnion	Higher Specialist Trainee, Neonatology
Andrew Wilkinson	Neonatologist, John Radcliffe Hospital, Oxford

This text was edited by Sam Richmond on behalf of the Newborn Life Support sub-committee.
Figures 5.1, 5.2, 5.3 & colour plates reproduced with permission of the Northern Neonatal Network who retain copyright.

Published by © Resuscitation Council (UK) 2011
5th Floor, Tavistock House North, Tavistock Square, London WC1H 9HR
Tel: 020 7388 4678 Fax: 020 7383 0773 email: enquiries@resus.org.uk website: www.resus.org.uk

Design & Print: TT Litho Printers Limited
Corporation Street, Rochester, Kent. ME1 1NN
Tel: 01634 845397 Fax: 01634 846807 Email: admin@ttlitho.co.uk Website: www.ttlitho.co.uk

Acknowledgements

This text started life in 1980 as a small booklet written to help midwives, nurses and doctors faced, for the first time, with a responsibility for the care of babies at birth. Early editions were written by Edmund Hey who, as a physiologist working with Kenneth Cross in the 1960s, was involved in much of the original research into the physiology of neonatal asphyxia and temperature control. They were written to complement a regional theoretical and practical course in newborn resuscitation in the Northern Health Region of the United Kingdom. The booklet remained a locally written text, though with considerable national and a small international distribution, through a number of editions published by the Northern Neonatal Network. The fifth and final edition appeared in 1996. The working group is grateful to the Network for permission to reproduce their physiological diagrams. Dr Hey retired from his post as consultant neonatologist at the Princess Mary Maternity Hospital in Newcastle upon Tyne in 1994 and died in 2009.

ILCOR: We also would like to acknowledge the inspiration and constructive challenges afforded by regular meetings and conversations with Jeffrey Perlman, John Kattwinkel and all the members of the neonatal section of the International Liaison Committee on Resuscitation (ILCOR) over the past ten years. Any reader interested in exploring the evidence behind the various recommendations made in this and other texts on the topic of neonatal resuscitation are urged to access the worksheets constructed during the most recent ILCOR assessment of evidence.[142]

Those who access the ILCOR consensus document via the Circulation website will notice a number of superscript codes – e.g. NRP014B – next to the headings addressing each specific question in the neonatal section (part 11). The number refers to the specific question and the suffix A, B or C on the same number denotes worksheets dealing with the same question but by different authors. Clicking on one of these will take you to the relevant worksheet giving that author's overview of the evidence and a detailed literature review of the published papers considered during the discussions leading to the final consensus document.

The URL is: http://circ.ahajournals.org/cgi/content/full/122/16_suppl_2/S516
(last accessed 01/12/2010)

The worksheets at the AHA journals website include the worksheet author's name and the comments of that author on the various papers reviewed but omit the abstracts of those papers. More complete versions of the worksheets which include the abstracts (but not the worksheet author's name) can be obtained via the ILCOR website. The URL of this website is: http://www.ilcor.org/en/consensus-2010/worksheets-2010/ <http://www.ilcor.org/en/consensus-2010/worksheets-2010/> (last accessed 22/01/2011)"

Cover photograph: This shows the scene a few minutes after a normal delivery. The father is cutting the cord while the mother gets ready for skin to skin contact. Compare the colour of the parents' hands to that of the baby. The cyanosed appearance of the baby is entirely normal at this early stage.

The Newborn Life Support course

The Newborn Life Support (NLS) course has been developed, under the auspices of the Resuscitation Council (UK), to provide clear practical instruction in resuscitation of babies at birth. It is designed for all health workers, regardless of their discipline or status, who may be called upon to resuscitate a newborn baby. The course is supported by the Royal College of Midwives, the British Association of Perinatal Medicine and the Royal College of Paediatrics and Child Health.

Aim of NLS

▶ **To give those responsible for initiating resuscitation at birth the background knowledge and skills to approach the management of the newborn infant during the first 10-20 minutes in a competent manner. The course concentrates on the effective teaching of practical airway management and ventilatory support.**

Learning outcomes

Having read the manual and completed a Newborn Life Support course you should:

1. Have sufficient background physiological information to understand the processes underlying apnoea, bradycardia and poor condition at birth and to grasp the principles of an approach to resuscitation at birth of such infants. These principles emphasise the overriding importance of airway management and lung aeration and the limited role of drugs.

2. Have had some practical experience in appropriate handling of the equipment used in resuscitation.

3. Have learnt fundamental skills in the management of the newborn airway including strategies to help in situations where the initial attempt at lung aeration is unsuccessful.

4. Have performed the following skills on manikins:

    - Airway management and lung aeration
    - Direct laryngoscopic inspection of the oropharynx
    - Chest compressions
    - Umbilical venous access

These are taught and assessed during the skill stations.

5. Have practised the immediate management of newborn emergencies in simulations and should appreciate the importance of communication and teamwork. This is assessed in a formative way during the simulation session followed by feedback with advice on areas for improvement.

6. Have demonstrated the core skills of airway management of a newborn infant in a test situation using manikins, and have shown that you know what steps to take if initial attempts at management are unsuccessful.

7. Have developed a framework for succinct recording and effective communication of important details of the baby's condition at birth and the response to resuscitation.

8. Have practised the skills and developed an approach to newborn resuscitation which, with further mentored clinical training, will permit achievement of clinical competence.

2 The size of the problem

Resuscitation, or should that be "assisted transition"?

In adult medicine the term 'resuscitation' is usually used to describe the urgent application of ventilation, chest compression, and often defibrillation, to an apparently lifeless adult. Yet almost every discussion of this topic in the paediatric literature starts with the unreferenced assertion that "resuscitation" is *necessary* in 6 to 10% of births. The need to apply both ventilation *and* chest compression to an apparently lifeless baby at birth is a rare event, occurring in about 1 in 2000 deliveries in countries with highly developed health care.[208] In the neonatal context it is clear that the term 'resuscitation' is often used somewhat loosely.

Some babies are clearly severely unwell at delivery and are unarguably in need of urgent attention to vital functions and this might legitimately be described as resuscitation. However, this is not the usual experience of an attendant called to help a baby at delivery. In most cases what is needed is assistance in achieving the transition from placental to pulmonary respiration. This is particularly true of the preterm infant.

Given that neonatal resuscitation is rarely defined in any detail, the frequency it is actually needed is difficult to determine. Furthermore, the fact that a baby *received* resuscitative measures at birth does not mean that the baby *required* such measures to ensure survival. A study at one hospital showed a fall in intubation rate from 7% to 1·5% following a change in policy which had resulted in fewer deliveries being attended by a paediatrician. One interpretation of this might be that a major risk factor for intubation at birth was the presence of a paediatrician.[99]

Information from Scottish hospitals shows that in the 1980s between 8 - 12% of babies born at a major hospital in Edinburgh were intubated at birth compared with between 1·5 - 2% of those born at a comparable hospital in Aberdeen.[81]

Perhaps the best information available on the *need* for resuscitation rather than its use comes from a study in Sweden.[138] All 100,000 births in the country over a year were studied. A standard approach was taught in Sweden advocating mask inflation initially with progress to intubation only if mask inflation was not successful. Amongst babies weighing 2·5 kg or more, only about 10 babies per 1000 received mask inflation or intubation. Of these babies 8 per 1000 responded to mask inflation and only 2 per 1000 seemed to require intubation at birth.[138] This conclusion is supported by a much smaller UK study involving about 18,000 deliveries at one hospital over 4 years which found that only 4 babies per 1000 over 37 weeks gestation were intubated in the last year of the study.[4] Though overall perinatal mortality figures are lower in Scandinavia than the UK, the birth weight specific perinatal mortality rates of the two populations are very similar.[109]

The equipment available for mask inflation 30 years ago was unsatisfactory, and lack of confidence in this method was widespread, which probably explains the high intubation rates at that time. When masks specifically designed for positive pressure ventilation were introduced in the mid 1980s[137] it was not surprising that it took a little time for this scepticism to disappear. These new masks, when used correctly, are able to aerate the lungs effectively and the perceived 'need' for intubation at delivery in the UK has fallen considerably in the past 10 years.

Which deliveries should be attended by a trained resuscitator?

Many labour ward policies suggest the need for a trained resuscitator to attend a delivery is judged by how the mother is to be delivered. A typical policy might demand attendance at all sections, all breech deliveries, all multiple deliveries, all instrumental deliveries, all preterm deliveries, all fetal distress and all meconium staining. Such a policy would involve attending more than 30% of deliveries and would not eliminate the need for urgent calls to resuscitate babies found to be unexpectedly unresponsive at birth.[145] A more logical approach would be to relate the need to attend a delivery to the presumed condition of the baby.

One study reported the efforts of paediatricians to reduce an attendance rate of 39% of deliveries to 25%.[99] Despite attending 39% of deliveries there were 20 further deliveries (1·5% of deliveries) where help was apparently required but had not been expected and this proportion neither increased nor decreased when new policies were introduced.

Whatever guidelines are used some babies will be born who unexpectedly require resuscitation. It is therefore important that everyone who takes on the responsibility of delivering babies should be trained in resuscitation at birth.

Why babies are different

CHAPTER 3

Objective

▶ **This chapter defines resuscitation and points out some of the essential differences in approach required when dealing with babies at birth.**

Introduction

Generally resuscitation is required when either breathing is interrupted, the circulation fails, or both. The immediate interventions required to aid recovery from this situation are generally termed resuscitation. Babies are not only smaller than adults but also different, and need resuscitation for different reasons. A different approach to the resuscitation of a baby or small child is therefore necessary from that adopted with a collapsed adult.

Adults

In adults collapse is usually a primary cardiac event, most commonly due to myocardial infarction, pulseless arrhythmia, or both. Breathing then stops because oxygen is no longer being delivered to the respiratory centre in the brain stem. The resuscitator therefore has to mimic the action of both the heart and the lungs in the hope of preserving flow of adequately oxygenated blood to the heart and brain. This is done using chest compressions interspersed with lung ventilation usually referred to as cardiopulmonary resuscitation or CPR. Having established a rudimentary circulation of oxygenated blood the problem with the heart has then to be diagnosed and treated. This usually requires a defibrillator, or occasionally, drugs. Throughout the time taken to do this an oxygen supply to the brain must be maintained using CPR.

Babies

Being pushed forward through the birth canal is a hypoxic experience for the fetus, because respiratory exchange via the placenta is interrupted for the 50 - 75 second duration of the average contraction. Though most babies tolerate this well, some do not and these few may require help to establish normal breathing at delivery. Thus, in newborn babies the problem is always initially a respiratory one.

The heart of the newborn baby can continue functioning for 20 minutes or more despite anoxia, during which time neural mechanisms driving attempts at normal breathing, and the reserve system of anoxic gasping, will have ceased to function if they were unable to draw air into the lungs [see Chapter 5]. To resuscitate a newborn baby it is usually sufficient merely to aerate the lungs. The circulation is usually still functioning and will then be able to bring oxygenated blood back to the heart from the lungs, leading to recovery. In rare instances the heart may need a brief period of chest compressions before the circulation is restored but significant rhythm problems do not occur. Therefore drugs and devices needed to deal with the cardiac arrhythmias that dominate adult resuscitation are not necessary.

Babies are prepared for the stress

The newborn baby has evolved to undertake the strenuous passage through the birth canal and the newborn baby's brain can withstand lack of oxygen for much longer than an adult brain.

Babies' lungs are fluid filled at birth

The newborn lung is fluid filled at birth which makes the technique of initial lung aeration different.

Chest compressions are more effective in babies

The cartilaginous rib cage of the newborn and the larger size of the heart relative to the chest make chest compression much easier as well as more efficient.

The reason for chest compressions is different in babies

In adult resuscitation the most effective intervention is usually defibrillation with chest compressions being used to maintain a circulation to the brain and heart until such time as a defibrillator can be applied.

In babies the crucial intervention is to aerate and then ventilate the lungs. Chest compression is needed in a very few cases and then only to assist the heart in delivering oxygenated blood to the coronary arteries and the heart muscle.

Summary

▶ **Babies who need resuscitation at birth have a respiratory problem. Once air enters the lungs, the heart usually responds. It follows that the most important skill to learn is that of effective airway management and successful lung aeration.**

Objective

▶ **This chapter reviews the immediate management of newborn babies including the majority who require no resuscitation.**

Introduction

Most mature babies will breathe or cry within 90 seconds of birth, some others need a little assistance and very few need resuscitation, even after an operative delivery. However, every newborn baby should be individually assessed at birth. It is not necessary to spend time trying to remove small amounts of liquor from the mouth and nose because the average 3·5 kg baby will clear more than 100 ml of fluid from the lungs and trachea quite unaided in a matter of minutes.[20, 105] They do not need to be held head down, given oxygen or subjected to vigorous suction but they should be dried and wrapped in dry towels to minimise heat loss.

Pause to assess the baby before clamping the cord

In utero the fetus respires via the placenta. After birth this function is taken over by the lungs. Following *normal* birth a *gradual* transition from one method of respiration to the other occurs. This can take a few minutes to complete, though in most instances it happens very quickly. While this is happening redistribution of blood between the placenta and the baby is also occurring. If the placenta is still attached to the uterine wall, and if the baby appears well, then there is no need to interrupt this process.

It is recommended that the cord should not be clamped for *at least* one minute after the baby emerges.[142, 209] To prevent heat loss the baby can be wrapped, or at least covered, during this interval. Very early clamping can cause hypovolaemia.[125, 211] For a more detailed discussion of the timing of cord clamping see chapter 24.

Warmth

Keeping the baby warm is essential. Because of their small size and relatively large surface area babies can get cold very quickly. Ideally the baby should be born into an environment that is warm enough to allow the baby to maintain a body temperature within the normal range without effort. A wet baby rapidly loses heat and a small baby can quickly become dangerously hypothermic.[34] Babies subjected to cold stress in the period immediately after birth have a lower oxygen tension[173] and an increased metabolic acidosis.[56] There is evidence in animals that hypoxia, acidosis and hypothermia all tend to inhibit surfactant production.[59]

Methods of heat loss

Heat loss occurs by four different routes: Evaporation, convection, conduction and radiation. When the skin is wet with amniotic fluid, moisture quickly evaporates from the skin surface taking a large amount of heat with it as latent heat of evaporation. Draughts of air moving past the baby encourage this and also cause loss of heat by convection. Placing the baby on a cold surface such as cool mattresses or towels will risk heat loss by conduction. Finally the baby may lose heat by radiation from uncovered skin surfaces direct to cooler surfaces. In the newborn baby most heat is lost by evaporation and convection.

Preventing heat loss

There are several simple and effective ways by which heat loss can be kept to a minimum:

- Dry the baby and wrap in a pre-warmed towel to prevent evaporative heat loss.[86]

- Keep the delivery area draught free by keeping doors and windows shut wherever possible, to reduce heat loss by convection.

- If the baby needs attention place the baby on a warm mattress under a radiant heater to reduce heat loss by radiation and conduction.

Initial assessment

Allow the baby at least one minute to adjust before clamping and cutting the cord. During this time keep the baby warm and assess:

- Colour
- Tone
- Breathing
- Heart rate

The items are listed in this order because this is the order in which this information becomes available. Colour can be assessed as soon as you see the baby, tone can be appreciated as soon as you see and touch the baby, breathing can be noted almost as quickly and detection of heart rate requires a little more time.

Reassess heart rate and breathing regularly during any subsequent resuscitation, as these are the first to change and can be used to guide your actions.

Colour

Look at the colour of the trunk, lips and tongue.

Tone

Check whether the baby is well flexed with good tone or floppy like a rag doll.

Breathing

Look at the rate and pattern of respiration. Most babies start breathing regularly within 30 seconds of birth. In one national study in the UK over 75% of surviving babies established regular breathing by 60 seconds. However around 20% of otherwise normal babies took between 60 - 180 seconds to start breathing regularly.[26]

Heart rate

Listen for the heart rate with a stethoscope or feel for a pulse at the base of the umbilical cord. In an apnoeic baby the slow pulsation of the ventricles can often be seen lifting the chest wall. However, even in a healthy baby the cord does not always pulsate, nor does the rate of cord pulsation always reflect the true pulse rate. If you feel a normal heart rate of over 100 beats min^{-1} in the cord it suggests all is well. However, if you feel a slow heart rate or no pulse at all this may not reflect the true heart rate.[136] Check with a stethoscope or a pulse oximeter.

Interpretation

A baby who is breathing regularly, with a fast heart rate, who is centrally pink and who has good tone needs no further intervention (other than to maintain its temperature) and should be given to the mother.

A baby who is not breathing adequately, who has a slow heart rate or one who is blue-white or floppy should be dried and covered and, if the situation allows, placed under a radiant heat source, so that further actions may then be taken.

> **CALL FOR HELP IF YOU FEEL YOU NEED IT**

Parents

At delivery, do not take the baby away from the mother unless this is clearly necessary. Both parents may want to hold and examine their baby and, if the baby appears well, they should be encouraged to do so, once the baby has been dried, assuming the delivery area is warm and draught free. This is also a very good time to initiate breast feeding. Mature babies are at very little risk of becoming cold while they remain in the warmth of their mother's arms, even if unclothed, if the mother and baby are protected from draughts by a blanket.[86] Respect the family's need for peace and privacy.

Early feeding

All babies experience a fall in blood glucose in the first few hours after birth. The lowest point of this fall can reach levels of 1 - 2 mmol/litre.[75] This level in adults would cause unconsciousness or even fitting but does not do so in term newborn babies because alternative fuels for the brain are usually easily available in the form of lactate and ketones. Lactate is relatively high at birth and falls in the first few hours, thus providing alternative brain fuel while blood glucose production from glycogen is set in train.[68] Within a few hours of birth most babies start to produce ketones which can also be used as brain fuel and which will be available for the first 72 hours or so while breast feeding becomes established.[68]

Preterm babies (less than 37 weeks) and babies who are wasted or small for gestational age are less able to produce this protective ketogenic response.[69] Infants of insulin-dependent diabetic mothers may have an apparently higher requirement for glucose.[100] Babies who get cold, and thus have to use energy to try to maintain their body temperature, will use up their fuel reserves more rapidly.

Examination

The baby should be briefly examined shortly after birth in the presence of the parents. This examination should check for any signs of cardio-respiratory distress, congenital anomalies or injuries that may have occurred during the birthing process. The baby must be kept warm during this process and all findings should be recorded in the baby notes. A more detailed examination will take place later.

Washing

There is no need to wash the baby at birth. Doing so makes the baby very cold unnecessarily.[86] Washing can easily wait a few hours, and preferably a day or two, until the baby's body temperature has stabilised.

Summary

▸ **Pause to assess the baby after delivery and, if all is well, wait for at least a minute before clamping the cord**

▸ **The importance of drying and covering the baby to prevent heat loss cannot be over emphasised.**

▸ **Do not take the baby away from the parents unless it is clearly necessary.**

5 Physiology of perinatal hypoxia

Objective

▷ **This chapter outlines some of the historical approaches to resuscitation at birth and describes the findings of the animal research on which modern resuscitation at birth is based. An understanding of this physiological data allows a logical approach to resuscitation to be developed.**

History

Until the late 1950's resuscitation at birth had never been subjected to systematic study. Numerous techniques such as intragastric oxygen,[2, 28, 30] the dropping of respiratory stimulant drugs on the tongue,[13, 35, 62] Eve's rocking method,[47, 48, 67, 71] hyperbaric oxygen[32, 80] and rapid hypothermia[29, 200] were widely advocated and employed with apparent success. Though therapeutically-induced hypothermia has recently been shown to be useful in reducing long-term neurological damage after significant asphyxia, it is of no help at resuscitation. All of these techniques are now discredited and several have been shown to be harmful. Yet more than 90% of the babies subjected to these treatments survived: vivid testimony to the fact that most babies at birth have remarkable powers of recovery.

We now have a much better idea of what happens when mammals are subjected to acute hypoxia during birth, thanks to the work undertaken by Geoffrey Dawes in Oxford,[37] Kenneth Cross in London,[33] and a number of other neonatal physiologists,[60] and a much better idea how to respond logically and effectively. Most of what we now know about the subject was learnt between 1957 and 1967 - a decade that witnessed a complete transformation in the way newborn babies were resuscitated.

The use of mouth-to-mouth resuscitation was first made respectable by Safar in 1958,[160] and the complementary technique of closed-chest cardiac compression was first described two years later.[98] Within a year there were reports of the latter technique being successfully used on a baby.[126] However, it took over thirty years for tracheal intubation to be widely adopted as it eventually was in the 1960's[65, 190] even though this approach had been strongly recommended by Flagg in America in 1928,[53] by Blaikley and Gibberd in England in 1935[19], and routinely used by Virginia Apgar around 1950.[6]

During normal labour, recurrent uterine contraction interferes with placental gas exchange resulting in a degree of fetal hypoxia. The process of labour stimulates production of adrenaline by the fetus[198] and thyrotropin releasing hormone by the mother.[175] This encourages the cells responsible for secreting lung fluid in the fetus to cease production and to begin to absorb fluid from the alveolar spaces, preparing the lungs for air breathing.

Fetal response to hypoxia

The diagrams below (Fig 5.1 to 5.3) show data derived from animal experiments outlining the response of a fetal mammal subjected to acute total hypoxia in utero. These data were obtained by opening the pregnant uterus of an animal in such a way as to avoid uterine contraction, then preventing the fetus from being able to aerate the lungs by placing its head in a bag of normal saline, and finally obstructing the fetoplacental circulation. It is likely that acute intrauterine hypoxia produces similar changes in the human fetus as all mammals studied have demonstrated an identical sequence.

At the onset of acute hypoxia the conscious fetus's breathing movements, driven by the respiratory centre, become deeper and more rapid. During this time the pO_2 falls rapidly and soon the fetus loses consciousness. Within a few minutes regular breathing movements cease as the centres responsible for controlling them are unable to continue to function due to lack of oxygen and the fetus enters a period known as primary apnoea. Up to this point the heart rate has remained much the same but soon falls to about half its normal rate, though the blood pressure is almost unchanged.

The initial fall in heart rate is probably a vagally induced event but this low rate is maintained because, due to lack of oxygen, the heart muscle has to function using anaerobic metabolism - a less fuel-efficient mechanism. This is possible in the newborn because the heart is packed with glycogen. Blood pressure is maintained despite a lower heart rate because vasoconstriction restricts flow to all but the most vital areas. At the same time the slower heart rate allows more time for the ventricles to refill in diastole and the stroke volume slightly increases. Overall, cardiac output drops but the fall is not as great as would be predicted from the fall in rate. By these methods circulation is maintained to the organs of the body that are most important for immediate survival but at a cost of further deterioration of the biochemical milieu due to the release of lactic acid as a by-product of anaerobic metabolism.

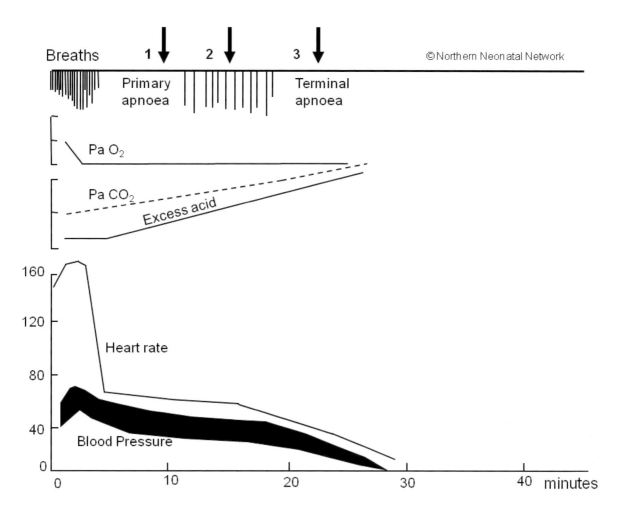

Fig 5.1 Diagrammatic representation of primary and secondary apnoea following the onset of acute total asphyxia at time 0

If the insult continues and the fetus is not delivered then, after a variable period of time, primitive spinal centres, released from suppression by the higher breathing centres, produce shuddering whole body gasps at a rate of about 12 min[-1].[37] A variable time may elapse before this unconscious gasping activity begins. Anaesthetics and drugs such as pethidine given to the mother can increase the duration of this primary apnoeic period but the length of the following period of gasping is then reduced.[122]

During this period of gasping some cardio-pulmonary circulation is maintained but if these gasps fail to aerate the lungs they fade away as increasing acidosis and hypoxia interferes with synaptic communication between nerve cells[61] and the fetus enters terminal apnoea. Soon the rapidly deteriorating biochemical milieu causes the heart muscle to cease to function effectively and, without further intervention, the baby dies. The whole process probably takes almost twenty minutes in the newborn human baby.[74]

A baby who is not breathing within a minute or two of birth could have reached one of the three points indicated by arrows in Figure 5.1. A baby born at the point indicated by

the first arrow will be perfectly able to 'resuscitate' itself provided the airway is clear. After a pause this baby will take the first of a series of gasps. If these gasps are successful in aerating the lungs then, because the circulation is still functioning, blood newly oxygenated by the aerated lungs will be transported to the coronary arteries and the heart rate will rapidly increase.

This, in turn, will mean that oxygenated blood is transported to the brain and the respiratory centre by the improving circulation. Once the respiratory centre is functioning again, normal regular breathing will start and gasping will cease. A similar sequence of events will follow in a baby born at the second arrow, though recovery may be somewhat slower.

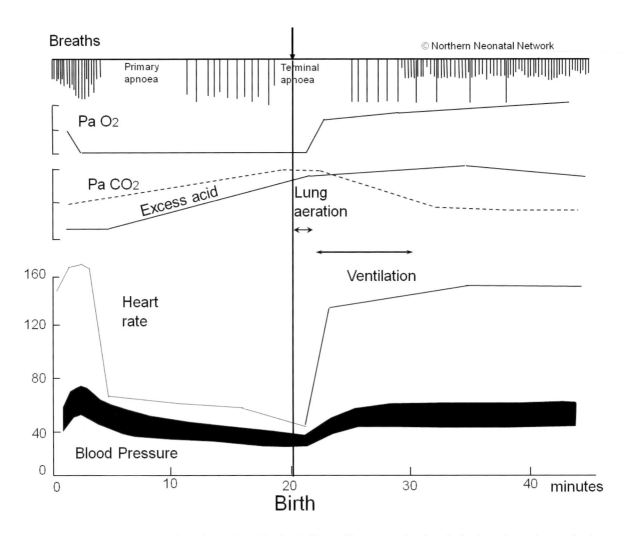

Fig 5.2 Diagrammatic representation of the physiological effect of lung aeration in a baby born in early terminal apnoea

A baby born at the point indicated by the third arrow will certainly die without intervention and may die despite it. However, effective lung aeration may be enough to produce a rapid recovery, provided the circulation is functioning sufficiently to bring some oxygenated blood back to the heart (Figure 5.2).

Unfortunately, it is not possible to tell at the time whether a baby who is not breathing at birth is in primary apnoea and about to gasp or whether it has already taken its last gasp in utero. It is reassuring to know, however, that almost all babies for whom help is called at birth will respond very rapidly once air or oxygen enters the lungs.

Figure 5.2 shows such a response to resuscitation from a baby in early terminal apnoea. A similar response would be expected had the baby been born in primary apnoea (arrow 1; Figure 5.1) but in that case one would expect few if any gasps following lung aeration.

However, in a few babies the situation may have progressed to a stage where the heart is no longer able to deliver oxygenated blood from the lungs to the coronary arteries despite adequate lung aeration with an appropriate gas. In this situation recovery may still occur in some cases if a brief period of chest compressions can

successfully deliver a small quantity of oxygenated blood to the heart and provided the heart is still able to respond as is illustrated opposite (Figure 5.3). This may need to be followed by a period of intermittent positive pressure ventilation until normal breathing is established.

As previously stated, it is impossible to tell at the time whether an apnoeic baby at birth is in primary apnoea and about to gasp or whether he has already taken his last gasp in utero and is now in terminal apnoea. A strategy needs to be developed which will cope equally well with either situation. Such a strategy is outlined in the next chapter.

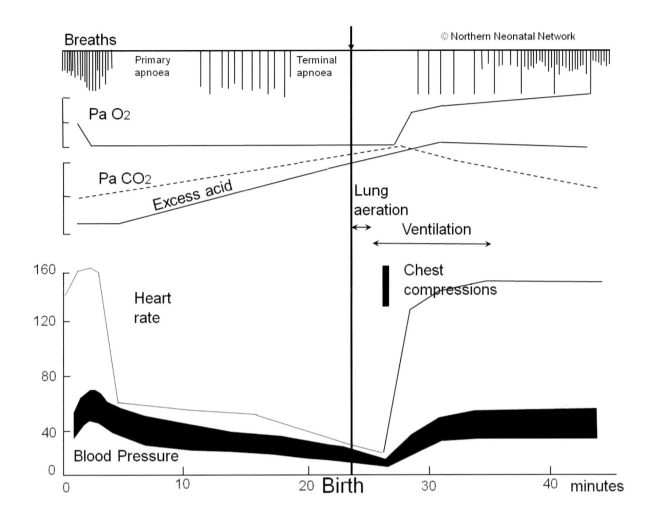

Fig 5.3 Diagrammatic representation of the physiological effect of chest compressions on a baby born in early terminal apnoea who does not respond to lung aeration and ventilation

Summary

There are three reasons why newborn babies can recover from periods of oxygen deprivation that more mature humans cannot endure:

▷ In response to hypoxia the baby conserves energy by shutting down the circulation to all but the most vital organs.

▷ After a latent period of so called primary apnoea, automatic, spinally generated gasping activity appears, while at the same time.....

▷ ....the heart of the term newborn baby is packed with glycogen which allows it to provide an adequate circulation in the face of considerable biochemical disturbance for a reasonably long time. This circulatory resilience is a feature of all mammals at birth.

CHAPTER

6 An overview of resuscitation

Objective

▸ **This chapter develops a logical approach to resuscitation for those few babies needing more than just gentle stimulation at birth. It is designed to be read once the preceding chapter on physiology has been thoroughly understood. It outlines the general approach to be adopted in resuscitation at birth. Practical details as to how each action should be done will be found in subsequent chapters.**

Introduction

Resuscitation is likely to be rapidly successful if begun before the baby has become so anoxic that all potential for respiratory activity has vanished.[42] Babies in primary apnoea can usually resuscitate themselves if they have a clear airway. This is why several useless methods, some of which were potentially harmful, were thought to be effective and were therefore relied upon for so long. As you do not know whether the apnoeic baby you are presented with is in primary or secondary apnoea you must develop a graded approach that will work in either situation. Always start by drying and covering the baby to prevent it from getting cold and then proceed as far as is necessary down the following list:

- Dry and cover the baby
- Assess the situation
- Airway
- Breathing
- Chest compressions
- (Drugs)

Dry and cover the baby

A wet baby rapidly loses heat, and a small baby can quickly become dangerously hypothermic.[34] Babies subjected to cold stress in the period immediately after birth have a lower arterial oxygen tension,[173] an increased metabolic acidosis,[56] and there is evidence in animals that hypoxia, acidosis and hypothermia all tend to inhibit surfactant production.[59] Unless obviously in need of urgent attention, the baby can remain attached to the placenta during this assessment. For a detailed discussion of the issues around cord clamping see chapter 24.

DO NOT LET THE BABY BECOME COLD DURING RESUSCITATION

Assess the situation

While drying the baby assess its colour and tone and then note the heart rate and whether the baby is breathing.

Airway

In order to breathe it is essential to have a clear airway otherwise air cannot be drawn into the lungs [see Chapter 8]. Babies in primary apnoea only require a clear airway in order to establish effective breathing (though most people would try to accelerate recovery by starting lung aeration). Provided the circulation is functioning, then oxygenated blood will be distributed to the heart and brain and the heart rate will rise.

Breathing

If the airway is clear and yet there is no effective breathing it is necessary to fill the lungs with air. First by inflation breaths to clear lung fluid, and then ventilation breaths [see Chapter 8]. In most cases the circulation is still functioning, in which case the first sign of effective oxygen delivery to the heart will be a rise in the heart rate. Breathing efforts may then improve at which point supportive ventilation may be discontinued. If the heart rate does not improve the most likely cause is failure to aerate the lungs and you should then check whether the lungs really have been aerated by checking for chest movement. Always ensure adequate ventilation before proceeding to chest compressions.

Chest compressions

If there is no rise in heart rate despite adequate ventilation, as judged by good chest movement, then the circulation may need assistance using chest compressions [see Chapter 9]. If correctly performed, this will bring blood from the lungs to the heart. *Provided the lungs have been aerated before chest compressions are begun* then the blood they cause to be returned to the heart will be oxygenated and this will allow the heart to respond with an increase in heart rate.

Drugs

In a few babies there may be no response despite good lung aeration, ventilation and effective chest compressions. This may be because of the effect of lactic acid accumulation and/or exhaustion of the limited glycogen stores in the heart muscle. In this situation reversal of the acidosis within the heart (with sodium bicarbonate), the provision of energy (with glucose) or stimulation of the myocardium (with adrenaline / epinephrine) may be successful, at least in theory [see Chapter 10]. If these drugs are used then central venous access via an umbilical venous catheter will probably be necessary [see Chapter 12].

Airway, Breathing, Chest compressions (and Drugs)

These steps must be tackled in this order. It will not be possible to aerate the lungs without a clear airway. Blood cannot be oxygenated unless air is delivered to the lungs. Chest compressions are pointless without oxygenated blood to move from the lungs to the heart.

Summary

▷ **Provided the airway is clear, most babies who are apnoeic at birth will resuscitate themselves.**

▷ **If resuscitation is required then the priorities - in this order - are:**

A - Open the Airway.

B - Aerate the lungs and Breathe for the baby.

C - Ensure an effective Circulation, with Chest Compressions if necessary.

D - Consider Drugs to achieve this if initially unsuccessful.

▷ **Don't let the baby get cold.**

▷ **Observe and record the sequence of events during resuscitation accurately.**

NLS

7 Resuscitation at birth

Objective

▶ **This chapter describes the process of resuscitation in more detail. It enlarges on the outline described in the previous chapter and aims to convey a feel for the timing of events in a typical resuscitation. For full details on the practicalities of airway management, circulatory support, umbilical catheterisation and the use of drugs the specific chapters on these subjects should be consulted.**

Preparation

If there is time:

- Make yourself known to the parents and explain why you are there

- Review the obstetric notes to identify any important factors

- Wash your hands, put on gloves and prepare the resuscitation area

- Make sure any heater is on and that doors and windows are closed

- Ensure there are enough warm towels (plastic bags for preterm babies)

- Check the gas supply and any delivery system - T piece/mask or bag/mask

- Ensure air/oxygen blender settings and pressure limits are set appropriately

- Check that a pulse oximeter and probe are available in case they are required*

- Check that the suction works and is set appropriately with the right type and size of catheter

- Ensure that airway adjuncts are available - oropharyngeal airways, laryngoscope / torch

- Check that equipment for intubation is available (if appropriate)*

- Check venous access equipment and resuscitation drugs (if appropriate)*

- Check the clock

*This level of equipment and expertise may not be available at home deliveries.

Consider

- **Do you need help?** - Senior support may be needed, especially for babies 30 weeks gestation or less [see Chapter 18]. Another pair of hands may be needed for twins, especially if born by caesarean section.

- **Is transport required?** - If the baby is likely to be very small or preterm then arrange to have a portable incubator and oxygen nearby for transfer. In the home, an ambulance may need to be called.

Anticipation can often prevent difficulties. If you are attending a birth at home there can be a considerable delay between asking for help and receiving it. It is better to have help arrive and not need it than to find you really need help which has not yet been summoned.

> **DO YOU NEED HELP ?**
> **DON'T BE PROUD**
> **ALWAYS ASK FOR HELP IF YOU EXPECT OR ENCOUNTER ANY DIFFICULTY**

After delivery

Drying and assessing the baby

- Start the clock or note the time of birth.

- For apparently well babies there is no need to rush to clamp the cord. Unless the baby is clearly in need of immediate resuscitation, wait for at least one minute from the complete delivery of the baby before clamping the cord. Keep the baby warm during this time.

- Collect the baby in a warm, dry towel.

- Dry the baby quickly and effectively. Remove the wet towel and wrap in a fresh dry warm towel. (For very small or significantly preterm babies it is better to place the wet baby in a food-grade plastic bag - and later under a radiant heater). [see Chapter 18]

- During this period it is possible to assess the baby and decide whether any intervention is going to be needed.

- *Then* clamp and cut the cord.

However, if the baby is thought to need assistance then this becomes the priority. In order to provide assistance the baby may need to be moved; which in turn may involve disconnecting the baby from the placenta. If the baby is limp or very pale, has a slow heart rate (less than 60 beats min[-1]) or is making no effort to breathe then transfer the baby to the resuscitation area.

Stimulation

The stress of delivery will stimulate the baby, as will the subsequent handling and drying. This is usually sufficient.

Initial assessment

Colour
Tone
Breathing
Heart Rate

Colour: Colour does not appear in the algorithm on page 16 because it is not as good a means of assessing oxygenation nor of how this is improving during resuscitation as was often previously thought.[132] However, it is mentioned here because it is still thought to be useful for assessing the initial condition of the baby at birth.

Babies in difficulties because of acidosis or serious blood loss will appear very pale at birth whereas the more normal colour is blue – see cover photograph. Very pale babies who remain pale after resuscitation may be hypovolaemic as well as acidotic.

Tone: Babies born well-flexed and with good tone are usually fine. A baby who is very floppy is unconscious and in significant difficulties. The tone of a baby is often clear from its posture but can also be rapidly assessed by handling the baby.

Heart rate: In healthy term babies the heart rate is usually greater than 100 min[-1] by two minutes of age but can be still below 100 min[-1] at three minutes in about 10%.[39] In well preterm babies this proportion is slightly greater.

Stethoscope: When first assessing the heart rate use a stethoscope. It is usually clear whether the heart rate is very slow (less than 60 min[-1]), slow (60 - 100 min[-1]) or fast (more than 100 min[1]). It is not necessary to count it with complete accuracy. The cardiac impulse can often be felt at the umbilicus. However it cannot always be felt, and the rate judged by cord pulsation, if slow, may not reflect the true heart rate.[136]

Pulse oximetry: Attempting to judge oxygenation by assessing skin colour is unreliable[132] but it is still worth noting the baby's colour at birth as well as whether, when and how it changes.

Using a pulse oximeter will allow accurate assessment of heart rate and oxygen saturation within about two

minutes of application [see Chapter 25]. Saturation levels in healthy babies in the first few minutes of life may be considerably lower than at other times.[38] In babies at birth the arterial oxygen saturation may be different depending on whether it is measured in areas supplied by blood leaving the aorta before or after the entry of the arterial duct; i.e. whether they are pre-ductal or post-ductal measurements. Measurements taken in the right arm are pre-ductal whereas measurements from other limbs will be post-ductal. The values quoted in the tables in this manual are all right arm (pre-ductal) values.

Values in the table below are taken from babies of **all** gestations in a study of over 450 healthy babies who received no resuscitation and no additional oxygen in the minutes immediately after birth. The data came from 308 term babies, 121 babies between 32 and 36 weeks gestation and 39 babies under 32 weeks gestation.[38]

The saturation levels listed in this table are deemed 'acceptable' in the sense that babies exhibiting these levels probably do not need any supplemental oxygen. However, babies whose saturation levels are significantly lower *might* warrant careful supplementation. Babies with oxygen saturations of 95% or more do not need added oxygen.

Time from birth	Acceptable (25th centile) right arm saturation (%)
2 min	60
3 min	70
4 min	80
5 min	85
10 min	90

A pulse oximeter can be very helpful in giving an accurate readout of heart rate and also has the advantage of giving information on oxygen saturation. If you don't have a pulse oximeter, a stethoscope is the most reliable means of monitoring heart rate.

If a baby has reasonable tone, and otherwise appears well despite a slow heart rate, then it is reasonable to wait a minute or so, whilst ensuring that the baby's head is appropriately positioned (see below).

Breathing: Breathing usually starts spontaneously within a minute of birth and whilst apnoea on assessment may warrant action it is important to realise that some perfectly healthy babies can take up to three minutes to start breathing after birth.[26]

The baby may show normal regular breaths, irregular breaths, gasping (sometimes interspersed amongst more normal breaths), or breathing may be absent (apnoea).

NLS

Gasping breaths are usually accompanied by recession but recession is also occasionally seen with regular breathing, suggesting increased work of breathing. This may be due to partial obstruction of the airway or stiff lungs in premature babies.

If the baby has a good heart rate and is making good respiratory effort then no further help is required. Once wrapped, this baby should be given to the mother.

Airway opening manoeuvres

If a baby is not breathing adequately, or is gasping, then the first step is to open the airway. The airway may be obstructed if the neck is either too flexed or too extended or - in a floppy baby on its back - if the tongue falls back into the airway due to loss of pharyngeal tone [see Chapter 8]. These mechanisms are more likely to be the cause of an airway problem than any mechanical obstruction from blood, thick mucus, or lumps of vernix or meconium.

After opening the airway and stimulation some babies start to make satisfactory breathing efforts in which case continue to support the airway, and observe. Reassess the heart rate to ensure this is satisfactory. No other action may be required.

Meconium

Most babies born through meconium stained liquor have not inhaled any particulate material into the lower respiratory tract. If they have not done so as a result of anoxic gasping before birth they will only very rarely do so at birth.[49] Suction of the baby's airways on the perineum or routine suction after delivery are no longer recommended but if a baby is born floppy, unresponsive and covered in thick meconium the airway should be inspected under direct vision and the oropharynx cleared of material which might obstruct [see Chapter 19].

> ## SCREAMING BABIES HAVE AN OPEN AIRWAY
>
> ## FLOPPY BABIES – HAVE A LOOK

Inflation breaths

In order to clear lung fluid in an unresponsive baby, positive pressure inflations with a long inspiration time are required [see Chapter 8]. For a term baby, start at pressures of about 30 cm water[79] with inflation times sustained for two or three seconds.[197] Five such 'inflation breaths' should be sufficient to aerate the lung. Significantly preterm babies (30 weeks and below) may well respond to a lower initial inflation pressure of 20 - 25 cm water [see Chapter 18].[171, 179, 163] In all babies start any resuscitation with air.

Having given 5 inflation breaths - reassess to see if the baby has responded.

Reassess – has the heart rate improved?

Heart rate *is* increasing

If inflation breaths have aerated the lung you would expect the heart rate to increase within 5 - 10 seconds. This is one of the first signs that the baby is responding. If the heart rate is increasing rapidly then you can assume that you have successfully aerated the lungs. You then proceed as follows:

- **Ventilation support:** Following inflation breaths the baby may start breathing spontaneously. If this does not occur, gently ventilate the lungs at about 30 breaths min[-1] until the baby starts to breathe. If your ventilation is adequate the heart rate will remain above 100 beats min[-1]. If it falls below this it suggests that your ventilation is inadequate. Recheck the airway position and ventilation technique. Pressures of around 20 cm water and inspiratory times of 1 second or less are usually adequate for ventilation once the lung has been aerated.

- **Reassess - is there spontaneous breathing?** With continued support, breathing efforts will usually return. The manner in which these return is important. If the first efforts are gasping in nature, this would suggest that the baby *may* have been in terminal apnoea. It is important to record the sequence and timing of events. If the heart rate is satisfactory but no spontaneous breathing returns then you might consider other factors such as sedation, neurological issues or intrathoracic pathology. Remember, it is possible to make a healthy baby apnoeic by lowering the pCO_2 with hyperventilation.

Heart rate *is not* increasing

If the heart rate is not responding the most likely reason is that you have failed to aerate the lungs. Go back and check airway opening manoeuvres and repeat the inflation breaths. This is the time at which to consider using two-person airway support and other airway manoeuvres [see Chapter 8].

- **Reassess - is there chest movement?** In the absence of a heart rate response, seeing the chest move as you give inflation breaths is the only way to judge successful aeration of the lungs. Listening for breath sounds with a stethoscope can be misleading because of transmitted upper airway sounds. Chest movement may only start to occur after the first few (two or three) effective inflation breaths. Check for chest movement with further inflation breaths. If confirmed, move to chest compressions - immediately if there is no heart rate. However, if there is now a detectable heart rate one might consider ~30 seconds ventilation and then reassess.

- **Reassess - is the heart rate satisfactory?** If the heart rate remains slow or absent, despite adequate ventilation as shown by chest movement, then you need to give chest compressions [see Chapter 9]. Chest compressions should help to move oxygenated blood from the lungs to the heart and coronary arteries. The blood you move can only be oxygenated if the lungs have air in them.

- **Reassess - has the heart rate improved?** It is usually only necessary to continue chest compressions for about 20 - 30 seconds before the heart responds with an increase in heart rate.[141]

- **Consider drugs:** If the baby has subjected to severe hypoxic stress then these simple measures may not be enough to produce an increase in heart rate. In this situation it may be necessary to use drugs to alter the intracardiac milieu or to stimulate the heart. The venous access necessary to give these drugs is most easily achieved using an umbilical venous catheter [see Chapters 10 and 12].

- **Reassess - has the heart rate improved?** If the heart rate is still not improving consider other factors such as hypovolaemia, tension pneumothorax, diaphragmatic hernia or, rarely, complete heart block.

- **Reassess - should resuscitation attempts continue?** If there was no detectable heart rate at birth and still none by ten minutes of age, survival is unlikely and long-term serious neurological disability amongst the rare survivors is almost universal. It is entirely appropriate to consider stopping at this point [see Chapter 11].[142, 209]

  If the heart rate remains slow at 10 minutes and is not improving the outlook is still very poor but the situation is more complex and senior advice should be urgently sought.

Summary

▶ **Dry and cover the baby**

▶ **Assess the situation**

▶ **Airway**

▶ **Breathing – inflation breaths**

▶ **Chest compressions**

▶ **(Drugs)**

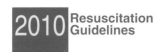 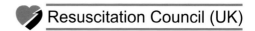

Newborn Life Support

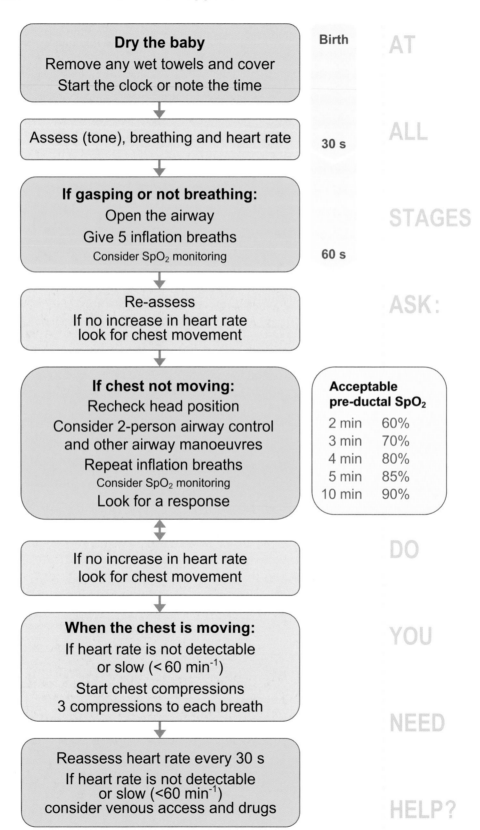

Dry the baby
Remove any wet towels and cover
Start the clock or note the time

Birth

Assess (tone), breathing and heart rate

30 s

If gasping or not breathing:
Open the airway
Give 5 inflation breaths
Consider SpO_2 monitoring

60 s

Re-assess
If no increase in heart rate
look for chest movement

If chest not moving:
Recheck head position
Consider 2-person airway control
and other airway manoeuvres
Repeat inflation breaths
Consider SpO_2 monitoring
Look for a response

Acceptable pre-ductal SpO_2

2 min	60%
3 min	70%
4 min	80%
5 min	85%
10 min	90%

If no increase in heart rate
look for chest movement

When the chest is moving:
If heart rate is not detectable
or slow (< 60 min^{-1})
Start chest compressions
3 compressions to each breath

Reassess heart rate every 30 s
If heart rate is not detectable
or slow (<60 min^{-1})
consider venous access and drugs

AT

ALL

STAGES

ASK:

DO

YOU

NEED

HELP?

Airway management

CHAPTER 8

Objective

▶ **This chapter provides the theory of airway management and positive pressure ventilation using a mask. The practical skills will be acquired through 'hands on' experience during the skill stations on the course, they will enable you to provide respiratory support to a baby at birth who is not breathing, or whose breathing is inadequate.**

Two key elements:

- Opening the airway
- Aerating the lungs - and then ventilating if needed

Opening the airway

In an unconscious baby lying on its back, the pharynx has a tendency to collapse and the tongue falls back obstructing the airway. This obstruction can be overcome by lifting the jaw (and thus the base of the tongue) forward. Two manoeuvres can be used to ensure an open airway in an unconscious baby:

1. Hold the head in the neutral position with chin support.

2. Move the jaw forward using jaw thrust.

MASK INFLATION CANNOT WORK

UNLESS THE AIRWAY IS OPEN

Head position

In most newborn babies the occiput is prominent and if the baby is placed on its back (supine) it causes the neck to flex. To correct this, place the baby's head in the neutral position with the neck neither extended nor flexed (Figure 8.1). If the baby is on its back on a flat surface then the neutral position can be easily achieved by placing a small (~2 cm thick) pad under the baby's shoulders.

Perhaps the most common reason for failure to open the airway is incorrect positioning of the neck - usually over extension.

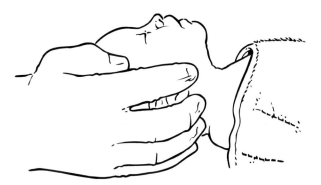

Figure 8.1 Hold the head in the neutral position.

Chin support and jaw thrust

In a baby with poor tone it will also be necessary to support the chin using a finger on the bony part of the chin near the tip (Figure 8.2). Avoid pressing on the soft tissue under the chin as this may push the tongue base backwards and worsen the situation. If the baby is very floppy it may be necessary to use one or two fingers under each side of the lower jaw at its angle to push the jaw forwards. (Figure 8.3).

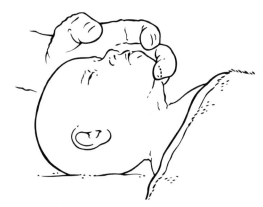

Figure 8.2 Chin support

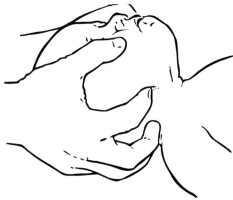

Figure 8.3 Jaw thrust

Aerating the lungs

Until the baby takes its first breath the lungs are filled with fluid. In fetal life the lung secretes large quantities of lung fluid which pass out into the amniotic cavity.[175] At birth all mammals studied so far have about 30 ml/kg of lung fluid ~ 100 ml in the average term baby. At the onset of normal labour various hormonal changes result in cells within the fetal lung switching from secreting to absorbing fluid.[172] A small amount of fluid, perhaps 35 ml or so in a term baby, is expelled via the oropharynx during the passage through the birth canal but once breathing starts about 70 ml[20, 172] is rapidly reabsorbed into the blood stream and the lymphatics within a few minutes.[105]

Babies who are born by section prior to the onset of labour will not have had the opportunity to 'prepare' their lungs in this way and this may go some way to explaining why such babies have a higher incidence of respiratory problems.[110]

Well babies can achieve lung aeration with their first breath using negative pressures of around minus 30 cm water, but frequently less than minus 20.[120] Well babies can achieve a resting lung volume of 15 to 30 ml with the first breath. Once a breath has been taken intrathoracic pressure is then often raised by crying to levels of 30 – 90 cm water. This presumably helps to drive lung fluid into the circulation during the first few breaths.

Babies needing resuscitation at birth need help in achieving a resting lung volume. If positive pressure ventilation is used then a relatively long inspiration time is required to aerate the lung of a newborn baby. When ventilating using positive pressure ventilation gas will not enter the lung until it reaches a pressure above the so-called 'opening pressure' of the lung. Theoretical calculations from measurements in isolated lungs as well as data from newborn babies would suggest that the opening pressure in babies apparently needing resuscitation is 15 - 30 cm water (1·3 to 2·8 kPa) with a mean of about 20.[21]

In term babies apparently needing resuscitation we therefore recommend using an inflation pressure of 30 cm water. Some suggest using a higher pressure because a higher flow rate will result. However, lung aeration depends on the volume of gas delivered which is a function of both flow and time. A lower pressure (if higher than the opening pressure) will be just as effective as a higher pressure, if applied for a longer time. Though a pressure of 40 cm water sustained for half a second can be effective,[192] an inflation pressure of 30 cm water applied for 2 - 3 seconds (and repeated five times) will adequately aerate the lungs of most babies at birth and this is the recommended approach.[73, 74, 197]

Facemask aeration and ventilation using a self-inflating bag as a source of pressurized gas is a skill that should be acquired by all involved in the care of the newborn. It can be difficult to do well, however, and requires practice.[128] Using a facemask with a T piece, a continuous supply of gas and a pressure-limiting device is generally felt to be easier, but requires a source of pressurised gas. This method was first described in 1913 and has been rediscovered on many occasions since.[72, 76, 88, 114]

The essential pre-requisites for both techniques are:

• A clear airway

• A good seal between the mask and the baby's face.

When aerating the lung consider the following:

Position the baby's head and jaw: Any baby hypoxic enough to require urgent resuscitation is likely to be unconscious and as limp as a patient under general anaesthesia, so the airway needs to be guarded and maintained. Use the airway opening manoeuvres described previously.

Clear the airway: The airway is usually clear but if in doubt consider gentle direct examination of the mouth and oropharynx using a laryngoscope. Do not blindly insert a suction catheter into the mouth. Stimulation in the region of the posterior pharynx and larynx should be kept to a minimum because it easily induces adduction of the vocal cords and profound vagal bradycardia (though it will have little effect in a baby in terminal apnoea).

Tracheal obstruction: Very occasionally the trachea may be obstructed by particulate matter aspirated before delivery or even after delivery. This can only be cleared by tracheal intubation and suction [see Chap 19].

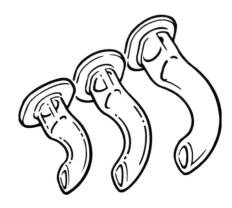

Figure 8.4 Oropharyngeal airways

An oropharyngeal airway (Guedel) should always be available and these are especially useful if there is some oro-facial abnormality affecting the airway. This can happen with a cleft palate - especially if there is micrognathia - or where the nasal passages are blocked or have not formed as in choanal atresia. Airways can also be helpful when you are having difficulty providing both jaw thrust and mask inflation on your own and help is not immediately available. Under these circumstances an airway of the appropriate size will perform the same task as jaw thrust - that is support the tongue forwards out of the oropharynx.

Choosing an oropharyngeal airway

When using an oropharyngeal airway it is important to choose the correct size. When held along the line of the lower jaw with the flange in the middle of the lips (immediately below the tip of the nose), the end of the airway should reach the angle of the jaw.

During insertion make sure that the airway slips over the tongue and does not push the tongue backwards into the back of the mouth. In babies and young children the airway is inserted in the same attitude that it will finally lie. It is not first placed upside down in the mouth and then rotated as is the usual method with adults.

Sizing the oropharyngeal airway as above is only approximate. Babies can vary in size from 500 to 5000g whereas there are only three sizes of oropharyngeal airway, 4, 5 and 6 cm. If the airway is too short the distal end will impact on the base of the tongue and may be occluded. If the airway is too long it may extend into the oropharynx below the tracheal opening and might obstruct the airway itself. The ideal length will reach just beyond the base of the tongue.

Choosing a mask

It is easiest to obtain a seal with a silicone mask with a broad, soft deformable sealing surface or flange. The soft flange of the mask is designed to be deformed by the baby's face; hold the mask against the baby's face and ensure an even pressure is applied around the circumference. Small babies need small masks.

The mask should cover the nose and mouth but should not extend over the edge of the chin and nor should it encroach on the orbits. Failure to achieve an airtight seal between the mask and the face is a common reason for failure of mask ventilation.

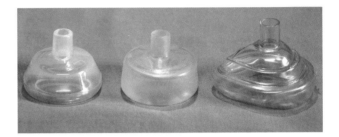

Fig 8.5 Suitable masks

1. Size the mask
2. Support the jaw
3. Re-check the airway position
4. Then give inflation breaths

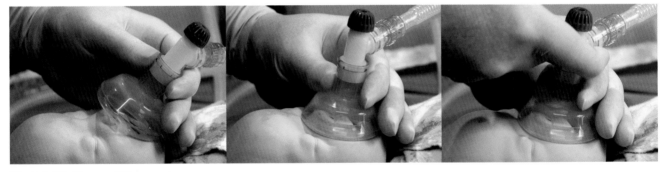

Fig 8.6 "Rolling on" the mask

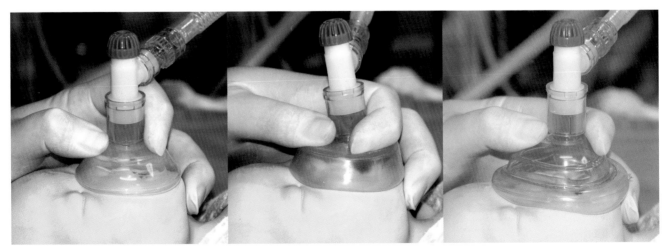

Fig 8.7 Suitable grips for the masks shown in fig 8.5

NLS

Give inflation breaths: Give five inflation breaths, sustaining the inflation pressure at about 30 cm water for 2 - 3 seconds with each breath. Too low a pressure is ineffective and too high a pressure can be dangerous.

The first two or three breaths will merely replace fluid with air without changing the volume of the chest. Therefore you would not expect the chest to move until the fourth or fifth breath. After the first half dozen breaths or so the lungs will be aerated and further ventilation can be managed with lower pressures (see below).

Lung aeration is more easily achieved with a constant-flow pressure-limited device, such as a T piece system, than a volume limited device such as a self-inflating bag. *Sustained* pressure is necessary to expand the lungs of the unconscious baby at birth, and this is less easily achieved with self-inflating bag-mask systems.[16, 52, 128]

Intubation can provide secure airway and frees the hands to concentrate on circulatory resuscitation if that is needed. However, the tracheal tube must be the correct diameter, the correct length, and securely fixed in the correct orifice. If any of these are not done properly then mask ventilation may be superior.

> **AERATE THE LUNG WITH FIVE 'INFLATION BREATHS' USING 30 CM WATER PRESSURE**
>
> **APPLIED FOR 2 - 3 SECONDS EACH BREATH**

Check for a response

If you have successfully aerated the lungs and if the heart can respond then you will detect an increase in the baby's heart rate. Therefore if an increase in the heart rate is detected you can assume lung aeration has been successful. If the heart rate does not increase this almost certainly means that you have not successfully aerated the lungs. In some cases, however, it may mean that you have aerated the lungs but the heart cannot respond.

If the heart rate does not respond to inflation breaths the only way to check that the lungs have been aerated successfully is to see the chest move in response to your inflation breaths.

No increase in heart rate? - look for chest movement

If you do not see chest movement after another five inflation breaths the most likely reason is that the airway is obstructed either because the head is not in the neutral position or because the jaw has not been drawn forwards. Two-person airway control or an oropharyngeal (Guedel) airway can be very helpful at this point. Only very occasionally is the airway blocked by mucus, vernix, blood or meconium. It is a mistake to assume that the airway cannot be blocked if there is no meconium present.

Use two people

It is much easier to give mask inflation with two people.[189] One person stands (or kneels) at the baby's head holding the head in the neutral position applies jaw thrust and concentrates on making a good seal with the mask. The second person occludes the T piece or squeezes the bag.

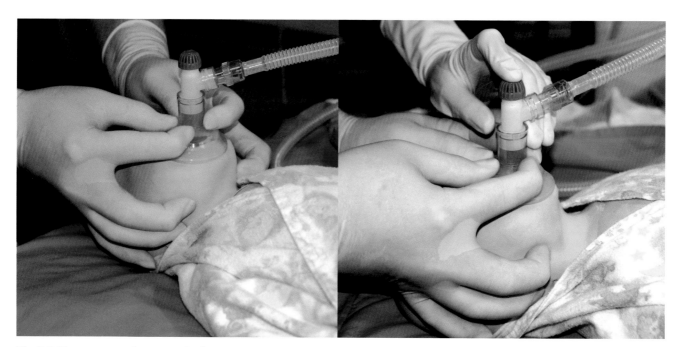

Fig 8.8 Two-person airway control

Equipment

NEVER CONNECT A BABY DIRECT TO A WALL OR CYLINDER FLOWMETER WITHOUT A SUITABLE BLOW-OFF VALVE IN THE CIRCUIT

T piece: A soft close-fitting facemask, a supply of piped air, and a suitable pressure release valve (preferably adjustable) are all that are needed (Figure 8.9). A small pressure dial in the circuit is a useful 'optional extra'. This can indicate that a good seal has been achieved if the needle rises to the set pressure. T piece circuits are also available that can provide PEEP [see Chap 25].

Self-inflating 'bag-mask' system: These can be used in much the same way where there is no piped gas, but are generally more difficult to use. Self-inflating bags are discussed in more detail in chapter 25.

Mouth to mask resuscitation

If you happen to have an appropriately sized mask and no other equipment then mouth-to-mask resuscitation is also very effective. It allows you to apply two-handed jaw thrust while at the same time holding the mask in place before applying your mouth to the mask. The pocket mask is designed for use in this way with older children and adults.

Mouth to mouth resuscitation

Mouth-to-mouth resuscitation is safe and it works. In larger babies mouth to nose resuscitation may be easier.[187] Of course, there are the usual concerns regarding transmission of potentially serious infection either to or from the baby; so use of appropriate equipment is always preferable. However, if equipment is not available it is certainly possible to resuscitate a baby at birth using this technique. Having dried and covered the baby just remember to:

- Keep the upper airway open using head position and perhaps jaw thrust, as described earlier.

- Cover the baby's mouth and nose with your mouth (or close the baby's mouth and use the nose alone).[187] Use long inflation breaths to start with.

- Watch for chest movement and allow a little time for the lungs to empty before inflating the chest again (20 - 30 breaths min[-1] will do).

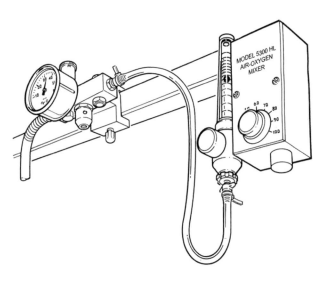

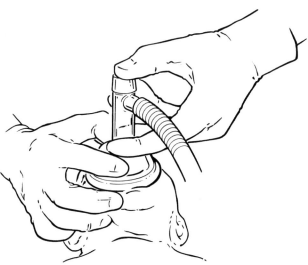

Fig 8.9 How to use a T-piece and mask

Summary

If the heart rate does not improve after five inflation breaths think:

▷ Is the baby's head in the neutral position ?

▷ Do you need jaw thrust ?

▷ Are you using a 2 - 3 second inflation time ?

▷ Do you need a second person's help with the airway ?

▷ Is there an obstruction in the oropharynx (laryngoscopy & suction) ?

▷ What about an oropharyngeal airway ?

Circulation

Objective

▶ **This chapter aims to provide an understanding of the thinking behind chest compressions and some of the important practical aspects of the technique. In other words, how it works, why you should do it, when you should do it, how you should do it and what to do if it doesn't work.**

Introduction

Before publication of the papers in 1960[98] and 1961[126] describing how cardiac massage could be done without opening the chest, it had only been infrequently tried at birth.[55, 64, 176] Soon closed massage was being widely adopted.[54, 176]

When is it needed?

The pulmonary circulation can be assumed to be at a standstill if the heart rate fails to accelerate once the lungs are aerated at birth.[37, 74] The cardiac impulse may or may not be audible or palpable, but there will be no pulsation present in the umbilical stump, skin circulation will be at a standstill, the blood pressure will be extremely low, and an ECG (if it were available) would probably show severe bradycardia– so called pulseless electrical activity.

Having established an airway and ensured that the chest is moving with ventilation, reassessment may show a persisting bradycardia. At this point it would be logical to provide chest compressions to help get the circulation going, providing you are certain lung aeration has occurred.

IF THE CHEST IS NOT MOVING THE LUNGS HAVE NOT BEEN AERATED

CHEST COMPRESSION IS USELESS IF THE LUNGS HAVE NOT BEEN AERATED

Before considering chest compressions make sure that you have managed to inflate the lungs. The only way to be sure is to see the chest move with each inflation breath. The baby who does not respond to lung aeration at birth is very rare[208] and the most likely reason for failure of the heart rate to increase after attempts at lung aeration is that you have not succeeded in aerating the lung. If using a mask check that:

- the head is in the neutral position and that the jaw is being drawn forward appropriately

- you have the right size mask and that there is a good seal against the baby's face

- there is a good flow of gas to your T piece (or that your self-inflating bag is working correctly [see Chapter 25])

- you are giving long inflation breaths

If you are using a tracheal tube check that it is correctly placed and that there is no leak around it.

Above all check that the chest is moving in response to your inflation or ventilation breaths.

GIVING CHEST COMPRESSIONS IS EASIER WITH HELP

CALL FOR HELP

How do chest compressions work?

Although it was originally thought that the heart alone was emptied of blood during chest compression, it is now considered more likely that compression of the entire thorax is important. During the compression phase, blood is squeezed from the chest by the increased pressure in the thoracic cavity. The blood flows forward into the arteries rather than into the veins due to the venous valves at the thoracic inlet and because muscular walls keep the lumen of arteries patent whereas the thin walled veins collapse. It is important that there is enough time in the relaxation phase to allow the chest to refill with blood.[159]

What am I trying to achieve?

Resuscitating babies at birth is different from resuscitating adults. In adult resuscitation you are usually dealing with a primary cardiac arrest and you need to keep oxygenated blood flowing to the brain and heart until the problem (e.g. arrhythmia, myocardial infarction) can be rectified. In the newborn baby you have a perfect physiological specimen that has been pushed beyond normal physiological limits. You are merely trying to re-establish effective heart pumping which should happen as soon as oxygenated blood reaches it; you can fully expect it to function virtually normally thereafter.

YOU ARE ONLY TRYING TO MOVE A FEW TEASPOONS OF OXYGENATED BLOOD FROM THE PULMONARY VEINS TO THE CORONARY ARTERIES

- A DISTANCE OF ABOUT 5 CM

Where should I press?

Compress the sternum over its lower third. If you press too high on the sternum the heart is not compressed; if you press too low, you risk damaging the liver. Place your thumbs on the sternum just below an imaginary line joining the nipples (Fig 9.1). Alternatively, locate the xiphisternum by finding the angle where the lowest ribs join in the middle and then prepare to compress the sternum at a point 1 finger's breadth above this. Compress the lower third of the sternum regularly by about one third of the depth of the chest, towards the backbone.[143, 119]

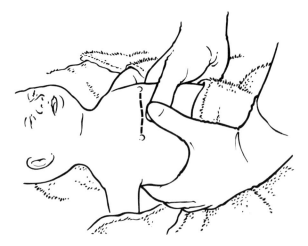

Fig 9.1 Two-thumb chest compression

Grip the chest in both hands placing the thumbs together at the front with the fingers over the spine. Your thumbs should be on the sternum and not on the ribs on either side.[36, 115, 180, 185]

Encircling the whole chest with both hands is the most effective method

If your hands are too small to encircle the chest then a less effective alternative[36, 115] to the above method is to press at the same point on the sternum with two fingers while the back of the baby is well supported (Fig 9.2).

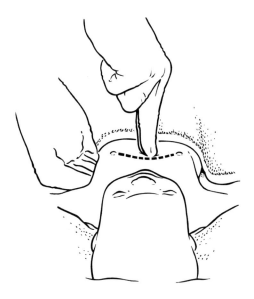

Fig 9.2 Two-finger chest compression

How deep should I press?

Try to reduce the antero-posterior diameter of the chest by one third with each compression.[119] Chest compression in the newborn does not cause rib fractures unless the baby has a severe bone disease such as osteogenesis imperfecta.[168]

How fast should I press?

Both the compression and the recoil are important. You are not trying to reproduce a normal neonatal heart rate of about 140 min[-1]. If you try to do so you will not produce effective blood flow because this technique is not as mechanically efficient as normal cardiac function. The rate you achieve is influenced by the chest wall compliance of the baby. Allow time after each compression for the chest to refill, by allowing it to re-expand fully. Remember, you are only trying to move oxygenated blood a short distance to restart the heart.

The current guidelines recommend compressions and ventilations in a ratio of 3:1 to achieve 90 compressions and 30 breaths (i.e. 120 events) in one minute.[142, 153, 209] In practice this can be difficult to sustain.[201]

CONCENTRATE ON GOOD QUALITY VENTILATION WITH GOOD QUALITY CHEST COMPRESSION

How long should I continue?

One would expect the heart rate to respond quickly to effective chest compressions, usually within 20 seconds.[141] Recheck the heart rate every 30 seconds or so to detect any response.

What if I get no response?

If you get no response to adequate chest compression combined with effective lung aeration and ventilation, the most likely reasons are myocardial dysfunction secondary to lactic acidosis, pulseless electrical activity (also known as electro-mechanical dissociation) or possibly exhaustion of myocardial glycogen. You will now need to consider using drugs.

Summary

▷ **Use chest compressions when there is a very slow or absent heart beat _and_ you are sure that _you have aerated the lungs_**

▷ **Press down quickly and firmly and then release.**

▷ **Aim to reduce the antero-posterior diameter of the chest by about one third with each compression.**

▷ **Allow the chest to recoil fully between compressions.**

▷ **Too rapid a rate gives the chambers of the heart no chance to refill passively after compression.**

▷ **Re-inflate the lungs after every 3 compressions.**

NLS

▶ **This chapter discusses the use of drugs in newborn resuscitation. Which drugs might be used, when they might be used, in what dose, and by what route they can be given.**

When are drugs needed?

Drugs should only be considered if, despite aerating the lungs, the circulation has failed and the heart does not respond to effective ventilation and good quality chest compressions. This is a very rare event, occurring in less than 1 in 2000 deliveries in a recent series of nearly 38,000 deliveries.[208] Though drugs have been used in this situation for decades there is very little evidence that they are effective and, though some babies appear to respond initially, the outlook is generally very poor.[166] Some studies report better results but careful reading suggests that drugs were sometimes used before the airway had been attended to and therefore presumably unnecessarily.[83, 129]

The most likely reason for chest compression failing to achieve a response is that it has been started before the lungs have been effectively aerated. Before using drugs check that the chest is definitely moving in response to inflation breaths either delivered by mask or tracheal tube and that the chest compressions are being performed appropriately.

> ## DRUGS ARE USELESS IF THE LUNGS HAVE NOT BEEN AERATED

How should drugs be given?

The circulation is not functioning and so drugs must be delivered as close as possible to the heart. This is best achieved by using an umbilical venous catheter (UVC).

Injections into a peripheral vein are unlikely to reach the heart when there is complete circulatory arrest. Direct injections into the umbilical cord vessels are useless for the same reason. Adrenaline can be given by the tracheal route,[106] though there are serious doubts as to whether it is effective in the newborn unless the dose used is significantly higher than that used intravenously.[142, 209] None of the other drugs mentioned below can be given this way. One very significant reason for avoiding

peripheral lines is that umbilical catheterisation is much quicker.

What drugs should I use?

Sodium bicarbonate

- **Preparation** 4·2% (or 8·4% diluted 1:1 with 5% or 10% Dextrose)
- **Dose** 1 - 2 mmol/kg (2 - 4 ml/kg of 4·2%)
- **Route** Umbilical venous catheter

If there is no effective cardiac output, or virtually none, then reversing intracardiac acidosis may be helpful. This is certainly true in animal experiments.[35] You are not attempting to correct the baby's metabolic acidosis, you are merely trying to improve cardiac function by improving the pH of the blood within the heart.

Give a small flush of 0·9% saline and a few chest compressions after giving any drugs and then assess the effect. An alkalising agent will normally produce cardiac acceleration within a couple of minutes if it is going to work. Bicarbonate must never be given down the tracheal tube.

Adrenaline (epinephrine)

- **Preparation** 1:10,000 (= 1 g/10,000 ml = 100 mg/L = 100 microgram/ml)
- **Dose** 10 microgram/kg (0·1 ml/kg of 1:10,000)
- **Route** Umbilical venous catheter (or via tracheal tube)

Animal evidence suggests that adrenaline cannot bind to its receptors at very low pH.[121] If there is no response to a dose of 10 microgram/kg it is arguably worth giving a dose of bicarbonate and then a further larger dose of adrenaline of 30 microgram/kg (i.e. 0·3 ml/kg of a 1:10,000 solution).

Unlike the other drugs mentioned in this section, adrenaline can be safely given down a tracheal tube.[150] However, if a standard 10 – 30 microgram/kg dose is given by this route it is not likely to be effective. A higher dose of at least 50 microgram/kg (maximum 100 microgram/kg) by this route might be considered but the safety and efficacy of such a dose has not been determined and use of standard doses via the intravenous or intraosseus route is preferred [see Chapter 24].

Dextrose

- **Preparation** 10% (= 10g/100 ml = 100mg/ml)

- **Dose** 250 mg/kg (2·5 ml/kg of 10%)

- **Route** Umbilical venous catheter

The heart cannot work without glucose and the glycogen stores present in the heart at birth diminish after birth. Dextrose can be tried if there is no response to adrenaline and bicarbonate. Ten percent dextrose is quite concentrated enough to supply a bolus of fuel to the heart. Subsequent symptomatic hypoglycaemia, if present, is better managed with an infusion of 10% dextrose rather than with repeated boluses. Dextrose must never be given down the tracheal tube.

Volume

- **Preparation** 0·9% Saline, (or a balanced salt solution)

- **Dose** 10 ml/kg initially

- **Route** Umbilical venous catheter

A bolus of about 10 ml/kg is usually sufficient to produce a response and can be repeated if necessary. If blood loss is the cause of the problem further transfusion with blood may be necessary later. Giving further volume to a severely compromised baby with a myocardium damaged by hypoxia is likely to do more harm than good. Giving large volumes (more than 40 ml/kg) of solutions high in chloride (such as albumin or 0·9% saline) can also exacerbate metabolic acidosis through hyperchloraemia.[167]

Summary

- **If bradycardia persists in the presence of adequate ventilation as judged by good chest movement, then start chest compressions.**

- **If bradycardia persists despite about 30 seconds of chest compression and adequate ventilation, insert an umbilical venous catheter and administer adrenaline and/or sodium bicarbonate, followed by further chest compressions.**

- **Volume expansion or dextrose may, rarely, appear to be needed.**

- **If lung aeration, ventilation and chest compressions are not working then the outlook, even with drugs, is very poor.**

CHAPTER 11 Babies who do not respond

Objective

▶ **This chapter looks at the possible reasons why a baby might not respond to the standard approach. If you are in this situation, call for help and remember that by far the commonest reason for failure is inadequate airway management.**

If the baby's heart rate doesn't respond after 5 inflation breaths, consider:

- Is the baby's head in the neutral position?

- Do you need a second person's help with the airway?

- Do you need jaw thrust?

- Are you using a 2 - 3 second inflation time?

- Is there an obstruction in the airway? (Laryngoscope and suction)

- What about an oropharyngeal airway?

Material blocking the trachea

Lumps of vernix, blood clot, thick mucus or particulate meconium, if large enough, can cause serious problems for the baby if inhaled into the trachea by gasping in utero. If you cannot aerate the lungs despite using a well fitting mask or tracheal tube, consider the possibility of impacted debris in the trachea [see Chapter 19]. Even if you cannot intubate look into the mouth with a laryngoscope and ensure that the oropharynx is clear.

The baby who remains blue

If the baby remains blue but has an acceptable heart rate, check for possible airway problems listed above. Keep ventilating and call for help. Other causes of continued cyanosis in a normal looking term baby are very rare. They include undiagnosed diaphragmatic hernia, intrapartum pneumonia or pneumothorax. It is rare for cyanotic congenital heart disease to be obvious this early though some cyanosis is present from birth. Use a pulse oximeter to check the oxygen saturation. Duskiness can be the first sign of persistent pulmonary hypertension which can easily spiral rapidly out of control if not recognised and treated quickly. You should be able to achieve 100% saturation in 100% oxygen if there is no right-to-left shunt.

CONTINUED CYANOSIS REQUIRES IMMEDIATE INVESTIGATION AND SENIOR HELP

Narcotics and naloxone

The baby affected by opiates given to the mother usually cries at birth, but becomes apnoeic when wrapped up warm and comfortable a few minutes later. The baby most at risk is one whose mother has had repeated doses less than 3 hours apart (the adult half-life), who has had doses IV rather than IM or who received the drug two or three hours before delivery. If a baby is apnoeic secondary to maternal opiates the urgent requirement is for lung aeration and subsequent ventilation. Only when the airway is secure, lung aeration has been achieved, the baby is ventilated or breathing and heart rate is normal, should naloxone treatment be considered. Naloxone is not an emergency drug.

Naloxone (200 microgram IM or 0·5 ml of 'adult' Narcan) given to the baby will reverse any opiate narcotic that may have been given to the mother.[123] Smaller doses (such as the 40 microgram ampoule of 'Neonatal' Narcan) will also reverse the sedation but the effect of this will only last a short time (20 minutes if given intravenously and a few hours if given intramuscularly) whereas the effect of pethidine (for example) can last for more than 24 hours in the newborn. Narcotics accumulate progressively in the unborn baby after administration to the mother.

Pneumothorax

If care is taken to limit the inflation pressure used then pneumothorax is a rare cause of problems at birth. It is not always necessary to drain a pneumothorax in the delivery room and directly aspirating the chest with a syringe and butterfly needle on the faint suspicion of a pneumothorax may well produce one.

However, in the very rare situation of a tension pneumothorax - suggested by a cyanosed baby with bradycardia who does not respond to ventilation and who has reduced breath sounds on one side – more urgent drainage may be needed.

Drainage can be performed by inserting a 20 - 23 gauge intravenous cannula (taking care to withdraw the needle once in the pleural space) into the fourth intercostal space in the anterior axillary line and aspirating any free gas using a syringe. If free air is present in a ventilated baby,

---

either keep aspirating or leave the cannula open until a definitive chest drain is placed. An alternative technique is to use a 23 gauge butterfly needle attached to a syringe. The butterfly needle will require manual support once inserted.

If possible it is best to transfer the baby to the neonatal unit and confirm the diagnosis by X-ray or by examination with a 'cold-light' before treatment.

The baby who is pale, shocked, dyspnoeic or hypovolaemic

This is rare, resulting from acute blood loss during delivery. It can occur with placental abruption, or after acute feto-maternal bleeding. Cutting through an anterior placenta during section can cause fetal blood loss. Pass an umbilical venous catheter and take a sample of blood for Hb (baseline) and crossmatching. Persistent bradycardia in these babies will often only respond to volume replacement which can initially be provided with 10 ml/kg of 0·9% saline or colloid solution (10 ml/kg is equivalent to giving a 70 kg adult a bolus of 700 ml of IV fluid). Later 20 - 40 ml/kg, blood will be required. Unmatched group O Rh negative blood is entirely appropriate.

A ruptured placental vessel (vasa praevia) can easily be missed as can blood loss into the baby's own abdominal cavity from trauma to the spleen or liver. Partial umbilical cord occlusion may close the umbilical vein but not the umbilical arteries (where the blood is at higher pressure) resulting in blood reaching the placenta but failing to return to the baby. A similar problem may follow shoulder dystocia, particularly if the cord is cut before the baby is extracted.[117] An umbilical venous catheter close to the right atrium is ideal for measuring central venous pressure. In the longer term the need for further blood can be assessed by watching for a progressive fall in haematocrit.

Hydrops fetalis

This condition is usually diagnosed by antenatal ultrasound and thus is unlikely to come as a surprise. The baby is pale and bloated with generalised oedema, ascites and occasionally pleural effusions. It may be necessary to tap the abdominal ascites (from the left iliac fossa so as to avoid damage to an enlarged liver or spleen) and apply an airway pressure of more than 30 cm water in order to achieve better diaphragmatic movement and lung aeration. Only if this does not work should you consider draining fluid from the chest. Pleural effusions may be present but only occasionally do they interfere with lung aeration.

Ascitic or pleural fluid is best drained with a relatively wide bore needle or cannula (e.g. 20 gauge) as this can be difficult through a narrower bore. In the very rare event that volume expansion is needed a crystalloid is preferred. Albumin or blood is relatively contraindicated because it

can raise the intravascular osmolality significantly resulting in rapid influx of tissue fluid and added myocardial strain. For the same reason it may be important to consider leaving a modest volume deficit after exchange transfusion.

When should you stop?

This question was addressed by the neonatal group on the International Liaison Committee on Resuscitation (ILCOR) in its most recent review of the published evidence in 2010.[142, 209] What little data there is on the outcome of babies with no detectable heart rate for 10 minutes suggests that they are highly likely to die or, if they should survive, to do so with severe neurological disability. It would therefore seem reasonable to stop resuscitation in a baby born with no detectable heart rate if the heart rate remains undetectable after 10 minutes.

However, whether or when to stop resuscitation in a baby whose heart rate is present but remains below 60 min[-1] after 10 minutes is much less clear and local senior advice should be sought.

There are also situations where the more pertinent question is, should resuscitation even be attempted. ILCOR has tried to address this question also. Clearly there are groups of babies defined by gestation, birth weight or the presence of specific congenital anomalies, that are associated with almost certain death or else rare survival but with very high morbidity and in these cases it is reasonable not to attempt resuscitation. However, what is perhaps more important is for local obstetric and neonatal teams to have developed a consistent approach to this problem in the light of local conditions.

Extreme prematurity

It is rare for a baby less than 500 grams at birth to survive, but many show signs of life after birth.[184, 205] It is dishonest and hurtful to brush aside such signs of life and classify the baby as stillborn especially when these signs have been witnessed by the family.

Most parents value having the opportunity to see and hold their dead or dying baby. Parents can readily understand that their baby is in the process of dying and can be grateful for the chance to share in this if reassured that the laboured gasps are not a sign of conscious pain or distress. They will want to be confident that the baby was assessed and that any chance of survival was not dismissed out of hand. It can be a comfort to stress that parent's love, care, comfort and warmth were the most important contributions to their baby's short life.

To handle this situation with sensitivity and skill calls for experience. Junior members of staff should not be left to face such situations without support. A framework for clinical practice endorsed by the British Association of Perinatal Medicine (BAPM) has been published.[203]

Each department should agree a guideline for planning and managing births at extremely low gestational ages. You should familiarise yourself with your local guidelines but if you are in doubt about whether to intervene you should start resuscitation and get a senior colleague to come and assist you immediately.

Definitions of live birth and stillbirth

UK: The legal definition of a live birth in the UK is *"a child born alive"*. Note that no gestational age is mentioned in this definition.

The legal definition of a stillbirth is a little more helpful and is *"A child which has issued forth from its mother after the 24th week of pregnancy and which did not at any time after being completely expelled from its mother breathe or show any other signs of life"*

Note that in the UK, babies born dead before 24 completed weeks of gestation are not registered as stillbirths but babies who are born alive at any gestation should be registered as live births.

World Health Organisation: The World Health Organisation (WHO) definitions are a bit more informative. The WHO definition of a live birth is *"the complete expulsion or extraction from its mother of a product of conception, irrespective of the duration of the pregnancy, which, after such separation, breathes or shows any other evidence of life, such as beating of the heart, pulsation of the umbilical cord, or definite movement of voluntary muscles, whether or not the umbilical cord has been cut or the placenta is attached; each product of such a birth is considered liveborn. Twins both born alive count as two live births but a child who dies from asphyxia caused by shoulder dystocia after delivery of the head but before delivery of the body is not a live birth."*

The WHO does not use the term stillbirth but refers to fetal death. A fetal death is defined as *"death prior to complete expulsion or extraction from its mother of a product of conception, irrespective of the duration of pregnancy; the death is indicated by the fact that after such separation the fetus does not breathe or show any other evidence of life, such as beating of the heart, pulsation of the umbilical cord, or definite movement of voluntary muscles."*

Summary

When babies fail to respond

▶ **If bradycardia persists in the presence of adequate ventilation as judged by good chest movement, then start chest compressions.**

▶ **Call for help**

▶ **Ensure that you are using all the skills you have learnt to keep the chest moving**

Also

▶ **Use chest compressions if the baby remains bradycardic**

▶ **Administer adrenaline and bicarbonate via UVC and consider volume**

▶ **Consider stopping resuscitation if the heart rate is still undetected after 10 minutes**

Umbilical vein catheterisation

CHAPTER 12

Objective

▶ **Inserting an umbilical venous catheter - When to do it, what you need in order to do it, how to do it and how to secure the catheter once you've done it.**

When to consider catheterisation

If the heart rate is still not improving despite good lung aeration, ventilation and a period of chest compression, then drugs or volume may be considered. Although umbilical vein catheterisation is seldom necessary in the emergency resuscitation of a baby at birth, it is a quick and effective way to gain access to the central circulation in a baby who has collapsed. It can be critically important to be able to give volume replacement or drugs, to transfuse a baby, or to sample blood from a baby who is peripherally 'shut down'. Trying to cannulate a peripheral vein is more difficult, slower and will be totally ineffective for delivering drugs to the heart when the circulation is absent.

Equipment

Immediate access to a sterile pack containing all the essential equipment makes rapid and reliable umbilical catheterisation much easier. A basic pack could usefully contain:

- scalpel and a straight edged blade (e.g. No 11)
- 5 French gauge end-hole umbilical catheter
- three-way tap and 5 ml syringe
- 2 pairs of artery forceps
- 1 umbilical vein probe, some sterile gauze squares, a cord ligature or tape

If this is a real emergency then there is no time for full aseptic technique, however you and an assistant should wear sterile gloves and observe universal precautions for your own safety.

Technique

Prepare the equipment. Fill a 5ml syringe with 0·9% saline and flush through a three-way tap attached to the umbilical catheter. Turn the tap to occlude the catheter to prevent air being sucked into the circulation should the baby gasp. Before you take a blood sample you have to suck back all the flush solution.

- **Tie** the cord ligature or tape loosely around the base of the cord. If a second twist is added to the tie (see Figure 12.1) then it will hold if it is necessary later to pull it tight. The arteries are unlikely to bleed though bleeding from the vein is likely. However, arterial bleeding may follow recovery.

- **Cut** the cord 2 cm from the skin with a clean stroke of the scalpel. A sawing action causes 'teeth' at the vessel edge making catheterisation difficult.

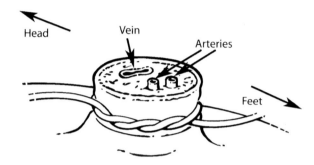

Fig 12.1 Identifying umbilical cord vessels

- **Identify** the umbilical vessels (Figure 12.1). There are usually two arteries and one vein; occasionally only a single artery is present. The vein travels 'north' from the umbilicus as the ductus venosus immediately beneath the anterior abdominal wall, passing through the liver to join the hepatic and portal veins then joining the inferior vena cava and entering the right atrium. The arteries are branches of the iliac vessels and enter the umbilicus from the 'south'. When the cord is cut close to the skin the thin-walled vein is usually found somewhere in the upper right quadrant, while the two stiff, string-like, white and bloodless contracted arteries are usually found somewhere in the two lower quadrants. Be sure to identify all three vessels.

- **Grasp** the cord with the artery forceps near the vein. With a second clip grip one wall of the vein before gently inserting the catheter into the vein using fingers or forceps. Do not probe the vein without supporting it by its edge with forceps. The umbilical vein may need to be gently dilated using a probe or a closed artery clip but is often easily entered without this.

- **Advance** the catheter until some resistance is felt at the umbilical ring just below the skin. Apply gentle pressure until the catheter passes through. The ideal place for the end of the catheter is within the inferior vena cava just outside the right atrium. In an emergency it is sufficient to get the end of the catheter in a large vessel – in other words into a vessel from which it is easy to aspirate blood.

Draw back on the syringe and blood should flow back if the catheter is in the right place. If blood is not drawn back easily insert the catheter a little further or withdraw it slightly and try again. The first sample of blood can usefully be sent for pH, blood gases and haematocrit estimation.

Flush the catheter gently with saline when in the right place to avoid thrombosis in the catheter

Tape - In an emergency, tape the catheter in place with one piece of tape across the abdomen. However, attaching adhesive tape to the thin skin of a preterm baby is best avoided because, on removal, the skin can be damaged. An alternative method for more permanent fixation is shown in figure 12.2.

Give drugs and 'fluid volume' if required.

Whenever possible umbilical catheterisation is best undertaken as a sterile procedure, in a properly equipped, warm, treatment area after the airway has been secured, and the circulation restored.

Securing an umbilical catheter

On the very rare occasions when this is needed as an emergency at delivery it almost always involves a term or near term baby. Under these circumstances the priority is to secure the UVC as central venous access. This can be done by generously taping the catheter to the abdomen.

If there is more time, one simple way to secure an umbilical catheter is to put two silk stitches into the substance of the umbilical cord, tie these in place and cut them about two inches long. Line these ends up alongside the catheter, turn the catheter back on itself and tape all together such that the catheter is taped to the silk. The catheter is then held securely in place with no tape attached to the skin. If it is necessary to adjust the catheter length after checking the position of the tip by X-ray or ultrasound this can be easily done.

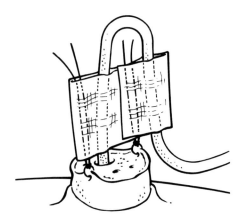

Fig 12.2 An effective system for more permanent fixation of umbilical catheters

Summary

▷ **If drugs are needed, the umbilical vein is the best route to use because it gives central venous access and inserting a UVC can be done rapidly in an emergency**

Tracheal intubation

Objective

▶ **This chapter discusses the practicalities of intubation. However, you cannot learn how to perform tracheal intubation from a book, a lecture, a manikin or a video. The best way is to be taught on an anaesthetised patient by an experienced practitioner.**

Why intubate?

Most babies who are apnoeic at birth respond to lung aeration with a facemask.[138] Intubation can occasionally be essential, for example, if the larynx or trachea is blocked with inhaled material. Intubation also provides a secure airway leaving the single handed operator free to concentrate on other things and in preterm babies it allows you to give artificial surfactant. Intubation, with the correct size tube, can also make the ventilation of abnormally stiff lungs easier. Surfactant deficient lungs, or 'dry' lungs following prolonged rupture of membranes (days or weeks) can sometimes be particularly difficult to aerate unless sustained pressures of 30 or even 35 cm water are used at first.[73, 192]

IT SHOULD BE POSSIBLE TO PLACE A TRACHEAL TUBE WITHIN 30 SECONDS

IF YOU FAIL TO DO SO, REVERT TO MASK INFLATION BEFORE TRYING AGAIN

When emergency intubation is necessary it can be assumed that the baby is already limp, unresponsive and unconscious. Tracheal intubation in such circumstances is not difficult, although it is not a skill that staff should be expected to display without prior supervised experience.[14, 15, 17, 135]

If a second person can check how long the procedure is taking and alert the operator if it is taking too long this can be helpful.[131]

Tube size

Use the largest suitable tracheal tube - a snug fit is important. Too small a tube may not allow you to aerate the lungs especially if they are stiff or full of fluid (as at birth). If the tube is too small gas will escape through the gap between the tube and the tracheal wall and, if the lungs are at all stiff, so much gas will escape through the leak that they will not be inflated sufficiently. This can easily be detected by listening at the mouth or over the neck with a stethoscope while inflating the lung. Bubbles may appear at the mouth and chest movement will be poor. If you have chosen the right size tube and you can hear a large air leak you have intubated the oesophagus.

Tracheal tubes are classified by their internal diameter (ID) in millimetres. If a parallel sided tracheal tube is used then most term babies will need a 3·5mm ID tube though a very large baby may need a 4·0 mm tube. Babies under about 1000g will need a 2·5 mm tube and those between about 1000 and 1800g may suit a 3·0 mm tube. Tracheal tubes from different manufacturers may have different wall thicknesses and though it is the internal diameter that is most important from the respiratory point of view, it is the outside diameter that determines whether the tube will fit snugly into the larynx of any particular baby. (For example 2·5 tubes can vary in external diameter from 3·5 to 4·1 mm and similar variations occur in other sizes)

Tube length

If the tube is in the trachea, but has been pushed too far down and into one of the main bronchi (not always the right) then chest movement will not be symmetrical. A number of algorithms exist for judging tube length by weight, head circumference or foot length but a well researched study has recently produced an algorithm based on gestation, which is the attribute most likely to be known at delivery.[91]

Oral tracheal tube lengths by gestation

Gest wks	ETT at lips (cm)
23 - 24	5·5
25 - 26	6·0
27 - 29	6·5
30 - 32	7·0
33 - 34	7·5
35 - 37	8·0
38 - 40	8·5
41 - 43	9·0

Confirming tube placement

After intubation, check that the tube is in the trachea:

- Check the heart rate - is it increasing?

- Does the exhaled carbon dioxide detector confirm intubation? [see Chapter 25]

- Listen at the mouth - is there a large leak?

- Look at the chest - are both sides moving equally?

- Listen to both axillae - is air entry equal?

If the tube is in the right place, the chest will move symmetrically as pressure is applied, and the heart rate will usually start to improve within about 30 seconds.

If the tube is not in the trachea there is likely to be a large leak around the tube which can usually be heard if you put your ear or a stethoscope to the baby's mouth while applying positive pressure to the tube.

> **ONCE YOU ARE HAPPY THE TRACHEAL TUBE IS IN THE CORRECT POSITION...**
>
> **SECURE IT**

Digital intubation

It is quite easy to intubate a newborn baby just using a finger in the mouth. This system was regularly practised in New Orleans for more than 20 years from the early 1940's.[206] Skilled practitioners were said to be able to place a tube in a baby with normal anatomy in 3 - 5 seconds using this technique (Figure 13.1). It is still the preferred system of intubation in some units.[66]

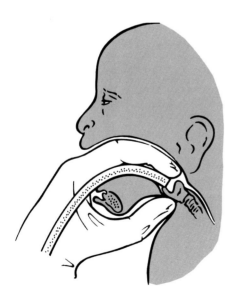

Fig 13.1 Digital intubation

This technique can be very helpful if you are faced with a child with facial or oral deformities that interfere with your ability to insert a laryngoscope or to see the larynx. Such problems can arise with severe Pierre Robin sequence (severe micrognathia often associated with a central cleft palate) and this technique can then be life-saving.

- Insert the index finger of your left hand into the baby's mouth, with its palmar surface sliding along the tongue. Use your little finger if the baby is small.

- Slide your finger along the tongue until it meets the epiglottis. This feels like a small band running across the root of the tongue.

- Slide your finger a little further until the tip lies behind and superior to the larynx and the nail touches the posterior pharyngeal wall.

- Slide the tube into the mouth between your finger and the tongue until the tip lies in the midline at the root of the distal phalanx of your finger.

- At this point place your left thumb on the baby's neck just below the cricoid cartilage in order to grasp the larynx between your thumb on the outside and your fingertip on the inside.

- While your thumb and finger steady the larynx against side to side motion your right hand advances the tube a short distance, about 1 - 2 cm.

- A slight 'give' can sometimes be felt as the tube passes into the larynx but no force is needed for insertion.

- When the tube is in the trachea the laryngeal cartilages can be felt to encircle it. If it has passed into the oesophagus it can be felt between your finger and the larynx.

Teaching and practising intubation

There are many plastic models of babies designed for teaching intubation but none provide an experience that is close to reality. Some are frankly misleading. This important skill is one that is probably best learned by practicing real intubation under supervision from an anaesthetist in an operating theatre.

The ethics of gaining this experience by intubating babies after death has been extensively discussed amongst the medical profession but only a few have written of their discussion of this topic with the public.[15, 23] It is a practice that should perhaps not be rejected out of hand; provided the family, having been sensitively approached by a senior member of staff, agree to it.

In one study 32 of 44 families consented to this teaching being done with their dead baby, five families agreed to this but refused permission for autopsy, four families agreed to autopsy but not to intubation teaching.[15] In the experience of the editor, some families have later expressed satisfaction that their tragedy has been turned to some good in this way.

Summary

▷ **Tracheal intubation is a valuable tool in the rare baby whose lungs cannot be aerated with good mask technique and in situations where ongoing ventilation is needed after the initial resuscitation.**

▷ **This skill is not taught or practised on the NLS course, but it is helpful for you to know when it will be needed and to have a clear idea of the process.**

Laryngoscopic intubation

Skill in responding to an emergency requiring intubation depends on the prior acquisition of good technique. Develop a standard, planned and structured approach from the start. Many have found the following approach useful.

- Position all the equipment you need close by and prepare a means of securing the tracheal tube once it is in place.

- Position the baby on a firm flat working surface with the neck partially extended. A roll of blanket under the shoulders of the baby may help. (Do not over-extend the neck as this will stretch the trachea and position the larynx very anteriorly, making it more difficult to see and also making it difficult to push the laryngeal opening into full view using external pressure on the larynx).

- Position the laryngoscope: hold the handle in your left hand while opening the baby's mouth. While looking down the laryngoscope insert it gently into the mouth. Be careful not to damage the gums.

- Position the tongue: In children and adults the usual approach is to insert the blade into the right hand side of the mouth and then to sweep the tongue into the left side of the baby's mouth by bringing the blade across into the centre during insertion. In newborn babies the tongue is usually relatively fixed in the floor of the mouth and it can be easier simply to slip the blade down centrally into the mouth over the tongue.

- Position yourself so you can see comfortably down the laryngoscope. If the blade is pushed in too far all you will see is the oesophagus (Figure 13.1A), you then have to withdraw the blade slightly to allow the larynx to drop into view from above (Figure 13.1B). Alternatively if the blade is not in far enough you may see little except the epiglottis (Figure 13.1C).

- Position the larynx. Once you have found the epiglottis, placing the tip of the blade at the base of the epiglottis where it meets the tongue (the vallecula) will bring the larynx into view from behind it (Figure 13.1D). Slight external downward pressure on the larynx may then help to bring the laryngeal opening into the centre of the field of view (Figure 13.1E).

- Position the tube: bringing the tip in from the right hand corner of the mouth and keeping the curve of the tube horizontal so you don't obscure your view of the larynx (Figure 13.1F). A stylet is usually unnecessary if you have everything properly lined up but may be helpful if it is difficult to direct the tip of the tube into the laryngeal inlet. If the cords are tightly adducted wait for them to relax - don't prod. (Reflex cord adduction proves that the baby cannot be in terminal apnoea.) Insert the tube 1 - 2 cm through the cords and no further (the marks on the tube will help to judge this).

- Secure the tube immediately, while you know it is still optimally positioned and note the distance inserted by noting the markings at the lips. Be careful, it is easy to allow the tube to go down too far. If you do, you risk ventilating only one lung.

- Aerate the lungs with 5 inflation breaths using a controlled inflation pressure of no more than 30 cm water sustained for at least two seconds, checking that the chest moves symmetrically.

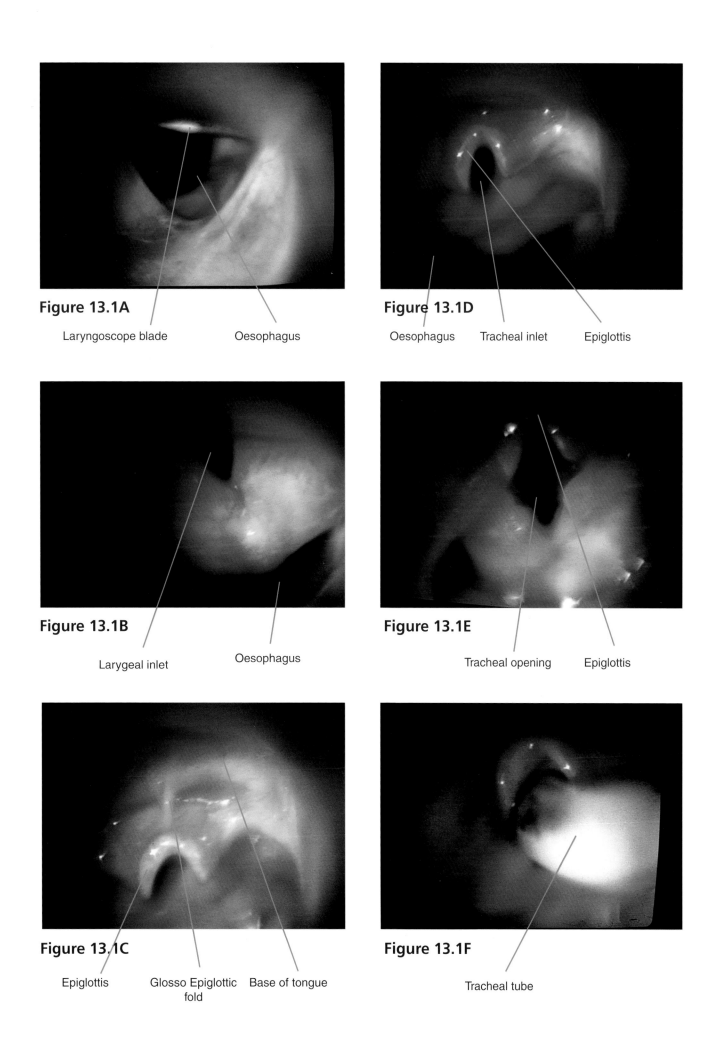

Figure 13.1A

Laryngoscope blade   Oesophagus

Figure 13.1D

Oesophagus   Tracheal inlet   Epiglottis

Figure 13.1B

Larygeal inlet   Oesophagus

Figure 13.1E

Tracheal opening   Epiglottis

Figure 13.1C

Epiglottis   Glosso Epiglottic fold   Base of tongue

Figure 13.1F

Tracheal tube

14 Immediate post-resuscitation care

This chapter and the following chapter attempt to summarise current opinion on further management after significant resuscitation after birth. The reader should be aware that whilst this represents current opinion, there is little objective evidence to support what is stated here.

Monitoring return of circulation and breathing

Behaviour during recovery from an asphyxial insult is a guide to the length and severity of the episode and should be monitored and documented carefully. Once the circulation is restored, anoxic gasping once every 10 - 20 seconds is almost always the first sign of recovery from true terminal apnoea. Ventilation should continue until normal regular breathing is established. Gasping may continue after normal respiratory activity appears. One measure of the anoxic insult to the central nervous system is the length of time from the return of a normal heart rate to the onset of normal regular respiration (with or without intermittent additional gasps).[28, 32]

Discriminating between primary and terminal apnoea

There is no instant way of determining if a baby is in primary apnoea and merely needs a clear airway or in terminal apnoea and needs active help. An Apgar score is frequently subjective and only tells you how unresponsive the baby is (but that may be a sign of shock, maternal sedation or immaturity rather than asphyxia), and a cord pH only quantifies acidosis at that moment. The only way to tell is to observe the sequence of events during recovery. The brain's response during recovery is the only index of how far the process had progressed.

As oxygen returns to the brain the various control centres recover. As the baby responds it will exhibit changes in behaviour in reverse order to that shown as it deteriorated, which should help to determine how far the baby had deteriorated. Babies who have been in terminal apnoea do not cough or gasp until the circulation is restored and always exhibit a period of gasping before normal breathing movements make their appearance.[1, 27, 74]

Continued airway support

If intubation has been necessary and if extubation is not appropriate then make sure that the tube is well secured and that there is good and equal air entry on both sides of the chest before transfer to the neonatal unit. Always incorporate a suitable pressure blow-off valve in the circuit between the source of gas pressure and the child. It is logical to use positive end expiratory pressure or PEEP during transfer, or at least as soon as possible. Never leave a small baby to breathe spontaneously against the resistance caused by a long narrow tracheal tube. Avoid over ventilation during transfer and try to avoid both hyperoxaemia and hypocarbia.[188]

Decisions about post-resuscitation care

Once the initial stabilisation phase is over, a care plan is needed which balances the need to keep the baby with the mother where possible, against the need for close observation and high dependency support in babies at significant risk of post resuscitation problems

When making decisions about post resuscitation care, the following factors need to be incorporated in a thoughtful risk assessment

- How great were the concerns of maternity staff about fetal wellbeing in labour?

- Do the cord gases suggest severe acidosis?

- Was the baby floppy, extremely bradycardic and without any respiratory effort at birth?

- How long did the baby take to respond to resuscitation?

- Were chest compressions used?

- Was gasping seen at any stage?

- Is the baby preterm or growth restricted?

- How is the baby now?: tone and behaviour, heart rate, breathing

Remaining with mother

If the decision is for the baby to remain with the mother, a clear plan of management, including early feeding and observation must be made and communicated to staff providing postnatal care. The use of structured early warning systems, with clear guidance on when to seek review will help to avoid any deterioration being missed.

Transfer to the neonatal unit

When moving the baby for transfer, keep the baby warm, maintain control of the airway and ensure intravenous lines are secured. Use appropriate transport equipment. If possible monitor oxygen saturation during transfer. Before leaving the resuscitation area ensure that the chest is moving and the baby remains pink. It is not easy to troubleshoot in a lift or corridor. Bear in mind the needs of the parents and make sure that they are fully informed of events and the reasons for transfer.

> ### ALWAYS LABEL THE BABY BEFORE LEAVING THE DELIVERY AREA

Record what you saw and did and speak to the parents [see Chapter 17].

Labelling the placenta for later examination

Detailed examination of the placenta, including a histological examination, can be very useful in elucidating the cause of problems in babies who are sick at birth or very preterm. Labelling the placenta and ensuring its transfer for pathological examination is often rewarding.

Kleihauer test

In cases where it is suspected that the baby may have lost blood it is useful to arrange for a sample of blood to be taken from the mother and examined for evidence of feto-maternal bleeding.

Summary

▷ **Remember that the baby who has been resuscitated is at risk of further deterioration and ensure that post resuscitation plans are made with patient safety in mind.**

▷ **Remember also that information from placental pathology and blood tests from mother may help in elucidating the underlying cause of the baby's problems.**

15 Later post-resuscitation care

Objective

> This manual is intended to deal with issues encountered during the first 10 - 20 minutes after birth. There are many textbooks dealing with subsequent intensive care. This chapter aims to give a brief summary of some of the most common problems which may occur after significant resuscitation. It is not intended to be a comprehensive list nor is it a complete review.

Later problems

A number of complications may occur after an anoxic insult. Though they may occur after a profound but acute insult, they are much more common after a less profound but prolonged insult.

Sepsis

Sepsis should always be considered as a possible underlying cause. It may be the primary reason for fetal distress. If this is a possibility, take appropriate cultures and start treatment. Consider preserving the placenta for later histological examination.

Respiratory depression

Some babies may need ventilation for a period after a hypoxic insult. Blood gases will need to be monitored and transfer to an intensive care unit will need to be arranged.

Blood gas monitoring: Beware over-ventilation. Respiratory acidosis can be treated by increasing ventilatory support. However, it is easy to over ventilate a baby with normal lungs and important to avoid hypocarbia and hyperoxaemia. Reducing the pCO_2 below 4 kPa reduces cerebral perfusion and is strongly associated with neurological damage.[101, 134] There is also evidence that hyperoxaemia is also associated with increased damage, especially if combined with hypocarbia.[95]

Oxygen saturation monitoring: Continuous monitoring of oxygenation is important. Persisting pulmonary hypertension, with blood by-passing the lung through the foramen ovale or ductus arteriosus, can rapidly become a serious problem if not detected and treated promptly. Appropriate ventilation and oxygenation may reduce the likelihood of this occurring. Early accurate diagnosis and treatment of this rare problem is likely to require echocardiographic investigation.

Monitor cardiac function

Post hypoxic transient cardiomyopathy is not uncommon and blood pressure monitoring is important. However, if myocardial function is compromised then it is unlikely to be appropriate to treat hypotension with a fluid bolus. Similarly premature babies may have impaired cardiac function due to the increased after-load on the heart which early birth entails.[96] Echocardiographic assessment of cardiac function can be very helpful in guiding appropriate use of inotropic support.

Metabolic acidosis

Virtually all babies who have descended as far as terminal apnoea will have a degree of metabolic acidosis. However, once the circulation is restored and respiration (or at least gaseous exchange) is established, this will be corrected over a period of several hours by the baby's lungs and kidneys. Though bicarbonate is very occasionally used during resuscitation if there is no cardiac output despite chest compressions it is hardly ever needed following successful resuscitation [see Chapter 10]. Slow partial correction of a metabolic acidosis is *occasionally* useful in certain circumstances, for example, in very immature babies, because a pH below 7·2 inhibits surfactant production. Even in these situations there is no need for rapid correction. Correction may also be appropriate as part of the treatment strategy if the baby is developing signs of persistent pulmonary hypertension with right-to-left shunting. In general, however, it is best to allow the baby to correct this by itself.

Consider therapeutic hypothermia

Sufficient evidence from randomised studies in babies has now accumulated for this treatment to be recommended in babies who have suffered asphyxia during delivery.[45] The techniques currently employed are those used in the various neonatal studies. However, the techniques are still evolving and in order to be able to refine these it is important to maintain a register of babies subjected to them.

In the UK this is done via the TOBY cooling register website (https://www.npeu.ox.ac.uk/tobyregister/) which also gives access to useful technical information. Therapeutic cooling should only be undertaken in centres with experience and the availability of EEG interpretation. Always discuss such babies with your network centres at the earliest opportunity.

Passive cooling: Once a decision has been made to offer cooling, if equipment for active cooling is not available, passive cooling can be started while arrangements are made to transfer the baby to a cooling centre. Passive cooling requires monitoring of rectal temperature but its use helps to avoid delays in starting treatment that would otherwise occur.[92]

Avoid hyperthermia: Hyperthermia, particularly when induced by external heating, is to be avoided at all costs in babies who have suffered perinatal brain injury.[24]

Convulsions: Amplitude integrated EEG or cerebral function monitoring, is helpful for obtaining evidence of cerebral depression. Anticonvulsants should be administered if there is seizure activity.

Monitor renal function

Temporary or more permanent interruption in renal function is often associated with intrapartum asphyxia. It may be appropriate to restrict total fluid intake to a minimum (perhaps 60 ml/kg per day) until renal function recovers. It will be necessary to adjust the frequency of antibiotic doses if renal function is reduced.

Urine output: Monitor urine output closely and do not be misled by urine already in the bladder at the time of the insult. Look at the early urine for blood, protein, cellular debris etc. Daily weighing is essential in monitoring fluid balance.

Sodium: Watch for hyponatraemia. Assess whether it is due to (a) oliguria and water retention, (b) cellular damage causing sodium redistribution within the body, or (c) renal loss of sodium, before attempting treatment. Measuring sodium and creatinine levels in both plasma and urine will allow you to calculate fractional sodium excretion which can also be helpful.

Glucose: Blood glucose levels may tend to be either too low or too high. Give a continuous infusion of dextrose and remember that, if using a low total fluid intake, it may be necessary to use a more concentrated solution to maintain blood glucose in the accepted normal range.

Summary

▷ **In the baby admitted to the neonatal unit post resuscitation monitor vital signs and biochemistry and intervene to maintain stability**

▷ **Remember sepsis and consider early antibiotics**

▷ **Consider therapeutic cooling in babies who are in very poor condition at birth and who demonstrate abnormal behaviour and tone after resuscitation.**

16 Long-term prognosis after significant resuscitation

Acute asphyxia

The prognosis for the full term baby subjected to sudden acute asphyxia (as a result, for example, of sudden immediately diagnosed cord prolapse or shoulder dystocia) can be very good, provided the episode does not last too long. Occasionally, however, even though the circulation is rapidly and effectively restored, cerebral function is very slow to recover.

The length of time it takes for reflex gasping activity to return gives some indication of the magnitude of the cerebral insult, but the length of time it takes for regular rhythmic (medullary) breathing to recover once the circulation is restored is a much more easily recorded event that gives a very good index of the severity of the cerebral insult.

Many of the babies who start to breathe again regularly within twenty minutes of the circulation being restored will recover completely but it is excessively rare for a baby who is still only gasping after thirty minutes to recover. The majority die within days and almost all the documented survivors have severe spastic quadriplegia and profound learning difficulties from widespread generalised death of brain tissue.[169]

Many healthy survivors show cerebral irritability for a few days and some have fits, but few show any other features and abnormal signs usually subside quickly.

The prognosis for the preterm baby of less than about 34 weeks gestation subjected to severe acute anoxia is more unpredictable however because there is a risk of secondary intraventricular haemorrhage or periventricular intracerebral haemorrhage and/or infarction after even a relatively brief asphyxial episode especially in the crucial period immediately before and after birth.

Ultrasound scans can give some indication of the position and size of the lesion but less indication of the amount of damage done and many major lesions cause surprisingly few symptoms at the time. While many children with major lesions on ultrasound turn out to be permanently handicapped the correlation between the initial appearance and the eventual outcome is seldom tight enough on its own to justify any decision to withdraw ventilatory support. Normal scans are not reassuring if the clinical picture suggests a poor prognosis.

Chronic asphyxia

Chronic asphyxia, can cause aspiration of vernix or meconium deep into the lung, can put the cardiac musculature under severe strain, can promote hypertrophy of muscle within pulmonary arterioles,[90] and can cause significant renal damage. It can cause serious cerebral ischaemia or haemorrhage, especially in the preterm baby, while in the mature baby ischaemia can also cause secondary cerebral oedema after a short, and deceptively encouraging, latent period.

Normal labour and delivery is a significantly hypoxic experience for the fetus. Both the fetus and the newborn baby withstand moderate chronic hypoxia (lack of oxygen) and asphyxia (lack of oxygen with a build up of carbon dioxide) remarkably well. However, really severe chronic asphyxia seems to be even more damaging than acute asphyxia. As an analogy, it is as though sudden total asphyxia stops the 'engine' abruptly whereas the chronic fuel starvation associated with severe chronic asphyxia 'wrecks the machinery' before the 'engine' finally fails.

The most worrying aspect of chronic asphyxia is the risk that secondary cerebral oedema and apoptosis associated with reperfusion injury will cause even more damage than the original period of asphyxia itself. In addition to this, although the fetal heart (with its large reserves of glycogen) is remarkably resistant to acute asphyxial stress, chronic asphyxia can so damage the myocardium as to cause a low cardiac output.[25, 182] This can have secondary consequences for other organs[141] particularly the kidney, which may develop 'pre-renal' failure due to poor perfusion. There may even be acute tubular necrosis.

An EEG can be helpful but requires expert interpretation to be useful. Recent large doses of anticonvulsants will make interpretation even more difficult. The long-term prognosis, however, depends largely on the depth of the post-asphyxial coma, the extent of any secondary cerebral oedema, and the severity and persistence of the seizure activity. A reasonably clear idea as to the extent of the problem should be obtainable within 36 - 48 hours of the original chronic asphyxial insult. A mild short-lasting state of hyperexcitability usually carries a good prognosis even if there is seizure activity but more severe symptoms can be associated with permanent handicap.

A quarter of the babies with hypotonia and suppression of normal primitive reflex activity (Grade II encephalopathy in the classification of Sarnat and Sarnat summarised on p 55), are handicapped, and the prognosis is even worse if there are fits. Most flaccid, stuporose babies (Grade III) die, and survivors are invariably handicapped.[155]

Longer term prognosis

From the prognostic point of view the initial state of the baby is less important than the speed with which the child responds to resuscitation once it is started. Even more important than the speed with which respiration and the circulation recover, however, is the speed with which the neurological signs improve. Fits are a bad sign and babies requiring ventilatory support for respiratory depression have an extremely bad prognosis, although it may be justifiable to offer continuing support where aspiration, pneumonia or seizures (and/or treatment thereof) jeopardise respiratory exchange.

All of the data used to produce the information in this chapter predates the use of therapeutic hypothermia. The publication of the Toby study in 2010 added a further set of results to the accumulating evidence in favour of early therapeutic hypothermia as an effective treatment for asphyxia at birth.[10, 45] It is possible that the introduction of this treatment to standard practice may alter the prognosis to some extent. However data published so far suggests that the effect is modest and apparently confined to those with a moderate degree of encephalopathy. For survival with a mental development index score of 84 or more, with normal hearing, normal vision and no cerebral palsy – all assessed at 18 months of age – the number needed to treat is 8.[45]

Other therapeutic strategies involving erythropoietin, magnesium sulphate, melatonin, topiramate and xenon ventilation remain to be explored.[103]

Summary

▸ **In the baby admitted to the neonatal unit post resuscitation monitor vital signs and biochemistry and intervene to maintain stability**

▸ **Remember sepsis and consider early antibiotics**

▸ **Consider therapeutic cooling in babies who are in very poor condition at birth and who demonstrate abnormal behaviour and tone after resuscitation.**

17 Communication and record keeping

Objective

▶ **When reading this chapter, remember that the incidents that trigger most complaints in the field of health care find their origin in poor communication.**

In an emergency, structured communication helps

Communication problems are a factor in up to 80% of adverse incidents or near miss reports in hospitals. This failure of communication is also evident when a newborn emergency occurs and a doctor, nurse or midwife summons senior help. The caller often fails to communicate the seriousness of the situation or conveys the information in a way that fails to ensure that the recipient appreciates the urgency of the situation. A well-structured process that is simple, reliable and dependable will enable the caller to convey the important facts, the degree of urgency and allow the recipient to plan ahead. Use of the acronyms SBAR (Situation-Background-Assessment-Recommendation) or RSVP (Reason, Story, Vital signs, Plan) can be helpful in planning effective, timely communication between individuals from different clinical backgrounds and hierarchies. Some are concerned that the acronym RSVP may be misheard as RIP if spoken aloud in the context of a serious emergency.

SBAR	Content	Example A	Example B
Situation	Introduce yourself and check you are speaking to the correct person Identify the patient you are calling about (who and where) State what you need	I am the senior midwife on the labour ward I am calling about Ms Smith There is cord prolapse and we are proceeding to immediate section	I am the senior midwife on the labour ward I am calling about baby Smith in room 5 The baby is grunting at one hour of age
Background	Important features of pregnancy and delivery Term or preterm Condition at birth and response to any resuscitation	Pregnancy has been normal Labour was normal until the membranes ruptured 5 minutes ago The umbilical cord has prolapsed	Pregnancy has been normal Delivery was by elective section for breech at 38 weeks The baby was in good condition at birth and did not need resuscitation, but has been grunting since 10 minutes of age
Assessment	**Undelivered mother** Progression of labour, CTG findings **Baby** Colour, Tone, Breathing, Heart rate	The cord is in the vagina It is still pulsating	Baby is pink in air, HR is >100, tone is normal, RR is 60 per minute with grunting
Recommendation	State explicitly what you want the person you are calling to do What by when?	Please attend theatre one immediately Please alert your seniors	I am not too concerned, but I would like you to review the baby within 30 minutes

Table 17.1

Written records

Accurate and comprehensive records are important, particularly in resuscitation at birth where records may be carefully scrutinised years later. Ideally, case notes should be prepared prior to the birth to allow for information to be collated in advance. If case notes are not available then the scraps of paper used to note down information during resuscitation may be attached to the case notes as they constitute a contemporaneous record of what took place.[41] Overall the record should 'demonstrate the chronology of events and all significant consultations, assessments, observations, decisions, interventions and outcomes.'[191]

Facts not opinions

Make an accurate written record of all that has happened as soon as possible afterwards. Consider very carefully the words used in such a record; and while you write imagine your words being read out to you in court. These records may assume considerable medico-legal importance later. Distinguish carefully between fact and opinion and consider very carefully the appropriateness of any adjective you plan to use. Record what you actually saw and did and make no assumptions as to causation. Facts relating to the birth (e.g. fetal bradycardia, non-reassuring cardiotocograph trace, low scalp pH) should be noted. Note the time of every event as accurately as possible. Words such as 'asphyxia', 'anoxia' and 'fetal distress' should not be used as they are impossible to define in this context.[165] The term 'flat baby' is particularly unhelpful whether spoken or written. Any reference in your notes to the obstetric handling of the case should be purely factual.

What to record

After any resuscitation the following information should be recorded:

- When you were called, by whom, and why

- The time you arrived, who else was there, and the condition of the baby on your arrival

- What you did, when you did it, and the timing and details of any response from the baby. Recording these in sequence is helpful.

- Whether the baby appeared atonic and areflexic at birth

- The baby's heart rate at birth and when it first exceeded 100 beats min[-1]

- The time when you were first certain that the lungs had been successfully aerated.

- Whether gasping respiration preceded the onset of rhythmical breathing, when gasping started and how long it lasted

- When the baby started to breathe evenly, regularly and effectively 30 - 60 times per minute (even if gasping is still occurring intermittently)

- The date and time of writing your entry followed by your name, your role and grade, your signature and your professional registration number

Blood gases

If there are concerns that the baby has been significantly compromised it can be helpful to obtain blood for measurement of pH, base deficit and lactate both from an umbilical artery as well as from the vein.[8, 63, 87, 199] It should almost always be feasible to pause after delivery to obtain these samples. Both arterial and venous umbilical cord blood gas status is easily determined if two clamps are put on a 10 cm segment of the cord a minute after birth and the isolated portion put aside. (Remember that in most cases it is appropriate to pause for a minute after full delivery of the baby before clamping the cord). Ideally these should be sampled and processed within 10 minutes. Blood pH estimation in samples from double-clamped vessels is reliable for up to 60 minutes but measurements of lactate are only reliable if analysed within 20 minutes.[8]

Communication with other professionals

Where a problem has been suspected antenatally or during labour, it should be communicated to the neonatal staff so that an appropriate plan of action can be drawn up. If the problem is diagnosed in the postnatal period then the general practitioner, community midwife, health visitor and other members of the primary health care team should be informed. The obstetrician and midwife responsible for the mother's care should also be informed. A telephone call may be appropriate to ensure a speedy exchange of information, rather than waiting for formally produced letters and memos. This can be followed up with a letter or note confirming the information. Conversations should be documented carefully and should include details of the persons concerned, the content of the exchange and the date and time.

Communication with parents

It is important to remember that the parents, however young or inexperienced they may be, are the people to whom all information about their child should be primarily directed. Ideally the information should be shared with both parents together and only with their explicit permission should information be given to others. Very occasionally circumstances may arise where information has to be shared with other family members first but this will be a very rare event.

NLS

The birth of a child is an exceptionally important event for parents and they will be extremely anxious if their baby receives resuscitation at birth. Always speak to the parents as soon as possible; before birth if circumstances allow and it is thought that resuscitation is likely to be needed. They will assume the worst even if their baby was only on the resuscitaire for a few minutes. Parents often fear that any baby receiving resuscitation is likely to be 'brain-damaged'. Let them see, touch and hold their baby even if the baby is going to the neonatal unit. However, don't let the baby get cold or cyanosed in the process.

Information given to parents or other family members about the baby and any possible outcomes should be objective and should avoid prejudging care. In particular, the person responsible for resuscitation is not usually in a position to make an informed comment on the management of the pregnancy or labour and delivery. This should be left for midwifery and obstetric staff to deal with. Any discussions with parents should be documented.

Stressful situations can inhibit the retention of information and the use of jargon may further complicate the situation. Check the parents' understanding of the information you have given them by asking them to explain what they think you mean. It is the job of professionals to explain effectively.

Language problems

Some parents may have difficulties with communication because of disability or language problems. In these situations interpreters may have to be used. Using other family members to translate important information is generally bad practice as they may not understand the information they are being asked to give, they may translate the information inaccurately and you risk breaching patient confidentiality. Any information communicated to the parents should be clearly documented and this record should include a note of the parents' reaction to the information and any questions that they ask.

When a decision is made not to resuscitate a baby, the parents should be closely involved and in agreement with the decision. The reasons for the decision should be documented, along with a record of the discussion with the parents and their reaction.

Summary

▶ **Communicate clearly and carefully with parents and other professionals. Make detailed notes of what you said to the family and when you said it.**

▶ **Keep clear, detailed, factual notes that are legible, timed, dated and signed.**

Preterm babies

CHAPTER 18

Objective

▶ **This chapter emphasises that most preterm babies, even those born at 30 weeks gestation or earlier, only need assisted transition from placental to pulmonary respiration - not resuscitation. Careful assessment followed by gentle, considered support rather than rapid action is what is usually required.**

▶ **The few that do really need resuscitation can be managed in a very similar way to term babies - with some minor adjustments.**

Degrees of prematurity

Epidemiologically speaking, term babies are those born after 37 completed weeks of gestation but the way this definition was arrived at can hardly be described as a triumph of the scientific method.[110] There are exceptions to every rule but, based purely on gestation, the probability of a baby needing significant assistance at delivery if born between 34 and 37 weeks gestation is little different from that of more mature babies. However, at 30 weeks gestation and below it is a different matter and every effort should be made to ensure that a senior person with extensive experience in dealing with preterm babies is present at their delivery. The remainder of this chapter is primarily concerned with these babies

Assisting transition rather than resuscitation

Most preterm babies are in reasonable condition at birth and are only in need of assisted transition, not resuscitation.[133] In other words they are fragile individuals needing careful handling and gentle support, not critically ill babies on the point of death. Provided they can be kept warm it is probably to their advantage to remain attached to the placenta for a period while establishing pulmonary respiration.[116]

Pause briefly to assess the baby before clamping the cord

In the very preterm baby this remains an area of considerable uncertainty. However, if the cord is still pulsating and the placenta is still attached to the uterus then the baby is probably still involved in placental respiration. Provided you have taken steps to keep the baby warm – see below – then there is probably no need to rush this to an abrupt end and a pause of a minute or so is reasonable. Use this time to assess the baby carefully. *If the baby's condition is satisfactory* then, once the baby has taken a few breaths or cord pulsation has ceased, the cord can be clamped and the baby moved to a resuscitaire.

Keeping the baby warm – plastic bags and radiant heat

Why? A rectal temperature of less than 35°C increases the risk of death in babies weighing less than 1500g and admission temperatures less than 32.9°C have been associated with more than 80% mortality.[169] Even a brief period of hypothermia is associated with impaired surfactant synthesis, impaired surfactant spreading within the lungs, pulmonary hypertension, hypoxia and coagulation defects. Acidosis and hypoxia further inhibit surfactant production.[59, 118]

How?
- **Environmental temperature:** Raise the delivery room or operating theatre temperature, ideally to at least 26°C for babies less than 28 weeks gestation.[93, 97]

- **Plastic bags under radiant heat:** There is now good evidence that it is easier to maintain the temperature of very preterm babies if they are placed immediately after birth, without drying, into a plastic bag.[112, 196] It is important to remember that the babies in these studies were also then placed under a radiant heater.

Some specially designed bags are available but any bags approved for use for wrapping food when cooked in a microwave may also be used. Obviously the face should not be covered with plastic but it is helpful to cover the baby's head with a hat. If you need access to areas of the baby within the plastic bag, a small cut can be made in the bag for this purpose. Once the baby is on the resuscitaire do not cover the plastic bag with anything else but leave directly under the radiant heater.

- **Plastic bags without radiant heat:** Presumably the main advantage of using a plastic bag is that it substantially reduces evaporation of liquid from the surface of the baby. Stepping into a large plastic bag up to your neck as you get out of the shower will have a similar effect but no-one would suggest that this will magically keep you warm if your surroundings are cold. Wrapping a baby in plastic and then placing the baby next to a warm object – such as its mother's skin – and covering both with a warm towel will probably keep the baby warmer than a similar baby not covered in plastic but the data is not available to prove this.

NLS

Helping to establish pulmonary gas exchange

The lungs are fragile: The lungs of preterm infants are more fragile and less compliant than those of term infants. At the same time the chest wall of the preterm infant is more compliant and less able to protect the lung against over-inflation. Over enthusiastic inflation of fragile lungs can predispose to serious inflammatory damage and long-term morbidity.[18, 89]

CPAP & PEEP from birth: If the baby is breathing spontaneously then applying continuous positive airway pressure (CPAP) will ease the work of breathing and help to prevent alveolar collapse in expiration. Many very preterm babies can be stabilised on CPAP at birth without any need for intubation.[124, 179] In the ventilated baby airway recruitment can be increased and end-expiratory airway collapse reduced by maintaining positive end-expiratory pressure (PEEP). Suitable CPAP levels are 5 to 8 cm water and 5 cm water for PEEP.

Gentle and gradual aeration: If lung expansion and positive pressure ventilation is needed at birth then the aim should be to *gently* expand the lungs of the infant so as to *gradually* maximise gas exchange surface area, to avoid over-distension while at the same time preventing collapse during expiration.

In experiments in preterm lambs use of large inflation volumes immediately after delivery caused significant damage. This damage was slightly less if surfactant was given before inflation. However, if large tidal volumes were only used after 10 minutes of more gentle ventilation much less damage was done.[82] This would suggest that a more gradual approach may be an advantage rather than aiming for rapid achievement of full lung inflation.

It is probably 'unreasonable' to attempt to fully inflate the lungs of the preterm infant too quickly, just as it is 'unreasonable' to expect a baby to achieve adult oxygen saturation levels immediately at birth.

Tidal volume: Significant damage can be caused by a small number of over-enthusiastic breaths. We can guard against this volume trauma to some extent by limiting the pressure applied to the gas in the airway but the best way is by limiting the volume change of the lung itself. This implies that the future may lie in measuring and adjusting the tidal volume administered rather than trying to estimate this clinically.[163]

If it is possible to include devices measuring expired tidal volume into equipment used for stabilising preterm infants at birth these should be used. Exactly what tidal volumes are safe and effective is not yet known but they should probably not be allowed to exceed 7 - 9 ml/Kg, which approximates the normal tidal volume of a healthy, spontaneously breathing term infant.[5]

Pressure and volume: Start with inflation pressures of 20 - 25 cm water. Even then it is still possible to inadvertently produce tidal volumes of 10 ml/kg. If these

pressures, applied for a sufficient inspiratory time, are unsuccessful higher pressures can be tried. Sustained pressures of up to 30 cm water may be required[73, 192] but should be avoided if possible to reduce the risk of lung injury in survivors.

The best guide as to whether satisfactory lung inflation is being maintained is a sustained increase in the heart rate. If the heart rate has increased satisfactorily then ventilation is probably adequate. Only if the heart rate has not stabilised should you seek to increase the degree of chest expansion. Clinical judgement is unreliable when assessing tidal volume based on chest excursion.[164] If significant chest expansion is easily seen it is likely that inflation volumes are too great and over-distension of the lung may be occurring.

If a preterm infant appears to need continued respiratory support then the baby should be attached to a modern ventilator as soon as possible and the settings adjusted to avoid excessive tidal volume.

> **Avoid over-distension of the lungs**
> **Start with pressures of 20 cm water**
> **and use PEEP**
> **Measure tidal volume if possible**

Intubation

Few preterm babies, even below 28 weeks gestation, *require* intubation at birth in order to survive. Some babies will also deliver unexpectedly outside the labour ward where the attendant may not only be inexperienced at intubation but may also have minimal equipment. It is safer to avoid intubation in such circumstances.[17] The normal algorithm should be followed, paying particular attention to drying the baby and keeping the baby covered and warm, and instituting good airway control and mask ventilation if necessary.

Intubation with the correct size tube will make the ventilation of abnormally stiff lungs easier. It will also allow administration of surfactant. Inflation pressures should be delivered in a controlled manner in order to avoid excessive inspiratory volumes, which might risk significant lung injury. Control of inspiratory pressure is most easily achieved using a T piece system rather than a bag-mask device. Ideally PEEP should be applied to reduce alveolar collapse in expiration and thus avoid the inevitable shearing forces which occur when collapsed alveoli and small airways are re-expanded.[171, 195]

Surfactant: For babies less than 30 weeks gestation there is a serious risk of respiratory distress syndrome and evidence that early prophylactic use of surfactant has advantages over rescue treatment.[181, 195] Early use of surfactant and CPAP can reduce the number of preterm babies needing ventilation.[195] Some units administer this in the delivery room, others on the neonatal unit.

Avoid both hyperoxaemia and hypoxia

Using a pulse oximeter to monitor both heart rate and oxygen saturation in these babies from birth makes stabilisation much easier [see Chapter 25]. Exposing babies at birth to high concentrations of oxygen can have significant adverse longer term effects.[152, 178]

The study reporting normal values for right arm (preductal) oxygen saturation levels in the first minutes after birth from over 450 babies contained data from only 39 babies born before 32 weeks gestation.[38] The 25th centile saturation levels in these preterm babies was very slightly lower than the same centile constructed from the data from all the babies in the study. The table below is the same as that in chapter 7 and shows the 25th centile values for all the babies in the study.

Time from birth	Acceptable (25th centile) right arm saturation (%)
2 min	60
3 min	70
4 min	80
5 min	85
10 min	90

For practical purposes the same values of 'acceptable' oxygen saturation can be used for both term and preterm infants. Remember, these saturation levels are deemed 'acceptable' in the sense that babies exhibiting these levels or higher probably *do not need* any supplemental oxygen. However, babies whose saturation levels are significantly lower might warrant careful supplementation.

And the rare preterm baby who actually needs *resuscitation*?

Rapid and accurate assessment of the condition of a preterm baby at birth requires some experience but, just as in term infants, preterm babies delivered in poor condition due to hypoxia or hypovolaemia require prompt resuscitation. If the baby does not have an effective circulation or if there has been placental abruption then there is unlikely to be any advantage in delaying clamping the umbilical cord.

Warmth: These infants should be placed in a plastic bag under a radiant heater immediately and be resuscitated as judged necessary using the standard approach to airway, breathing and circulation. The presence of asphyxia adds urgency to the need to establish effective ventilation and the situation is no longer one of encouraging gentle transition. Asphyxia, will continue until effective ventilation is established.

Lower inflation pressures: Start with 5 inflation breaths at pressures of 20 - 25 cm water. Then check the heart rate and - *if the heart rate is not improving*, ventilation pressures should be increased until visible chest expansion is identifiable.

Consider reducing ventilation pressures as soon as you achieve a response.

Although preterm infants at risk of RDS may benefit from surfactant replacement, this should not be considered a drug of resuscitation as a bolus of surfactant may briefly compromise ventilation before it becomes more widely distributed.

Summary

‣ **Most preterm babies need support and 'assisted transition' rather than resuscitation in the minutes after birth**

‣ **Plastics bags and overhead warming are the best methods for preventing hypothermia**

‣ **Establish oxygen saturation monitoring as soon as you can**

‣ **If the baby has satisfactory oxygen saturation and heart rate and is making regular breathing attempts try mask CPAP, starting with air**

‣ **If the baby does not breathe, begin with inflation breaths at 20 - 25 cm water, starting with air.**

‣ **Use the saturation monitor and adjust the air/oxygen blender to avoid hyperoxia and hypoxia**

Objective

When attempting lung aeration...

▶ **..if the heart rate remains slow, and the chest does not move then the AIRWAY is the problem.**

▶ **When more common causes have been ruled out consider tracheal obstruction even in the absence of meconium**

Tracheal obstruction

Tracheal obstruction only rarely occurs at delivery. However, it is very important to develop a logical approach to resuscitation and to bear this rare but important complication in mind. Reports of a recent court case concerning this complication are very instructive.[111, 113, 144]

A baby gasping in utero or during delivery can inhale debris deep into the trachea. This can then block the trachea, frustrating attempts at lung aeration. It is important to be aware that meconium is not the only substance that can do this. A blood clot, a lump of thick vernix or viscid mucus or any other particulate matter, if large enough, can cause obstruction in the trachea.

Aspirating the trachea

Material thick enough to cause airway obstruction cannot be sucked up any catheter small enough to be passed down inside a tracheal tube. The whole tracheal tube should be used as a suction device as illustrated in Figure 19.1. Otherwise use the widest bore suction catheter available – preferably a 12 or 14 French gauge suction catheter.

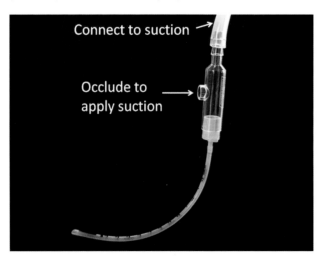

Connect to suction →

Occlude to → apply suction

Fig 19.1 With a suitable adaptor a tracheal tube can be used as a suction catheter

Meconium

The normal gentle 'breathing' efforts of a baby in utero are not sufficient to inhale particulate meconium in significant quantities. It is therefore reasonable to assume that if a baby has inhaled significant quantities of particulate meconium in utero then that baby has been gasping. In other words that baby has been asphyxiated to such an extent that it has passed through primary apnoea and into the gasping phase before delivery. If that is the case then the major determinants of the outcome for that baby are the circumstances and severity of the hypoxic insult that caused the baby to gasp rather than the meconium inhaled as a result of the gasping. Prolonged partial asphyxia can cause hyper-reactivity of the pulmonary vasculature and, in severe cases, excessive muscularisation within pulmonary vessels, resulting in persistent fetal circulation, pulmonary vascular necrosis and haemorrhage.[90]

Most babies born from meconium stained liquor have not inhaled any particulate material into the lower respiratory tract. If they have not done so as a result a period of anoxic gasping before birth they will only very rarely do so at birth.[49] Large, multi-centre randomised studies have shown that the previously advocated practice of aspirating the airways of the emerging baby before delivery followed by intubation and suction of the trachea after delivery – the so-called 'combined obstetric and pediatric approach' - is not effective and does not prevent the development of meconium aspiration syndrome.[193, 204]

Laryngeal inspection

If a baby born from within a sea of thick meconium is also floppy and makes no immediate respiratory effort, then it is probably reasonable to rapidly inspect the oropharynx with a view to removing any particulate matter that might obstruct the airway.

> **SCREAMING BABIES HAVE AN OPEN AIRWAY**
>
> **FLOPPY BABIES – HAVE A LOOK**

Summary

When attempting lung aeration...

▸ ..if the heart rate remains slow, and the chest does not move then the AIRWAY is the problem.

▸ When more common causes have been ruled out consider tracheal obstruction even in the absence of meconium

20 Birth outside labour ward

Planned or unplanned

Birth outside labour ward can be planned or unplanned. Planned home births usually involve low risk pregnancies delivering at term and a normal delivery is expected. For planned home births one can expect that the details concerning who is going to attend, when and how they will be called, what equipment will be needed, how it will be obtained, and what the backup arrangements are in case of emergencies have all been worked out in advance. However, if the birth is unplanned, none of these arrangements will have been made, the pregnancy may not be low risk and the baby may be preterm. This chapter will try to cover both situations with suggestions as to how to resuscitate the baby as safely and effectively as possible.

In the majority of situations where birth occurs outside hospital, the professional supervising the delivery is a midwife. The midwife's duty is to provide care to both woman and baby. While resuscitating the baby the midwife must be aware of the physical and psychological well being of the mother and at no time while resuscitating the baby should the mother be out of the vision and hearing of the midwife.

The maternity services strategy of the UK government places great emphasis on providing a choice of birth environments to meet the needs of mothers and their babies. This has resulted in increased numbers of births outside acute hospitals. A number of official documents have been drawn up, by government and other bodies, relating to and regulating this process.[156, 157]

Planned home births

Planned births outside hospital should be offered with clear referral and transfer arrangements in place in case of emergencies or complications. All NHS maternity care providers must ensure that community based facilities are *'fully equipped and staff have the skills for initial management and referral of obstetric and neonatal emergencies'.*[40] During the antenatal period the mother and her family should have been made aware of the on-call arrangements, the preparations to be made within the home, what equipment may be required and any transfer arrangements and procedures.

Environment

Temperature

Maintaining the normal temperature of the baby can more difficult outside hospital, but it is equally important. A suitable area for attending to the baby needs to be identified and prepared in advance. A firm, flat elevated surface area should be cleared and towels or substitutes made ready. Cover the baby's head with a hat and then, if appropriate, place the baby in direct skin to skin contact with the mother, or other warm adult body, under a towel or under clothing. Alternatively the baby should be dried and wrapped in *warm* towels or clothing.

Close the windows and doors to prevent draughts. Use stand-alone heaters if available. Consider the kitchen as the area for resuscitation and use radiators to heat towels. But be careful not to overheat them; test the temperature against the inner aspect of your forearm. Hot water bottles can also be useful but should never be put in direct contact with the baby – wrap them in a towel and check the temperature against your forearm.

Timing

Use your watch or a clock in the house – preferably one with a sweep second hand.

Equipment

Exactly what equipment should be carried for planned home births is a matter for local decision. Some equipment may be provided by the family. A minimum list is available through the Resuscitation Council (UK) website (www.resus.org.uk).

At birth

If possible two health professionals, at least one of whom should be a qualified midwife, should be present at birth. Tasks should be allocated depending on the situation and the skills of those available.

Detailed discussion of the midwifery and obstetric practicalities are beyond the scope of this text, but physiological management of the third stage is likely to be more appropriate in this situation. Active management of the third stage using syntometrine may delay attendance on the baby. If the baby is in difficulties then physiological management of the third stage may be more appropriate.

The resuscitation of the newborn in the home, as in any other environment, follows the standard algorithm.

Help

Within any locality where home births take place an agreed system of 'who should be called when' needs to be in place. In most cases help will be available via an emergency call for a paramedic ambulance but in more remote areas other means may be used. If the home does not have a functioning telephone then some alternative needs to be arranged.

Transfer

If a baby needed resuscitation at birth then transfer to hospital is advisable. If only one midwife is present then mother and baby should not be separated during transfer unless this is unavoidable. Ask the ambulance staff to increase the temperature in the ambulance prior to transfer. If the temperature is uncomfortably warm for an adult it will be about right for the baby.

If the baby is maintaining his airway well, then he can be transported held close to mother. However, if the baby requires support then special arrangements will be needed. Depending upon the locality this may require a neonatal transport team with a portable incubator. If a decision has been made to bring the baby into hospital whilst still resuscitating, then the stretcher is used as a base to resuscitate the baby and the environment should be as warm as possible. Remember to consider the safety of the whole team in this situation.

Unplanned births outside labour ward

Call for help early – you will almost certainly need it. Unplanned births are more likely to be premature or involving babies or mothers with health problems. An unplanned birth may occur anywhere a pregnant woman might be. The approach to resuscitation is the same anywhere but the availability of equipment, personnel and experience will obviously vary.

Birth in an ambulance

Stop the Ambulance

It is not possible to manage a birth safely in a moving ambulance. Ask the crew to stop the ambulance and increase the heating. One of the ambulance crew should make immediate radio contact with ambulance control who can relay the information to the nearest maternity unit or other centre.

Mother

Ask the mother to sit upright if she can as this will leave space to deal with the newborn. Leave the cord intact while resuscitation takes place. Leave the placenta to deliver physiologically after cutting the cord. Support the mother and **do not attempt to deliver the placenta** in transit. Observe progress of the third stage and watch for bleeding.

Baby

The baby should be resuscitated, if needed, in the standard manner. Once the baby is safely born, make sure he is kept warm, continue to make clinical observations and restart the journey. A baby in good condition can be given to the mother for skin-to-skin contact, or else wrapped and held by the mother.

Record keeping

Clinical records of delivery at home should be maintained in exactly the same way as they are for births anywhere else. Records should continue to be made during transfer.

Summary

In birth outside the hospital setting, take control of the environment and follow the same principles

- **Call for help early**
- **Dry, warm and cover the baby**
- **Assess**
- **Open the airway, use inflation breaths**
- **Chest compressions if no response**
- **Continue until help arrives or you are exhausted**

Objective

▶ **The Apgar score and Sarnat grading are common scoring systems used to classify babies at birth or soon after. Sarnat grading is used to grade encephalopathy, particularly if hypothermia treatment is being considered. Neither score should be recorded simply as a number. A detailed description of the baby is essential.**

Apgar score

This score has major limitations. It was originally devised for use as *'a basis for discussion and comparison of the results of obstetric practices, types of maternal pain relief and the effects of resuscitation'.*[6] It is of some use in categorising groups of babies, but of no use in the clinical management of individual babies.[7] Virginia Apgar, who was an obstetric anaesthetist, did not expect the score to predict mortality in individual babies but she did hope it might reveal a relationship between condition at birth and later neurological outcome.[7] In fact it does do this to some extent but it is very non-specific.

A recent large cohort study from Norway shows that babies with a very low Apgar score (3 or less at 5 minutes) have a 11% risk of showing signs of cerebral palsy (if they survive to one year) as compared with a risk of 0·1% for babies with a very high score (9 or more).[104] However, this tells us little about the cause of the cerebral palsy. Babies with low scores would include those with a longstanding problem prior to birth, those who had suffered a recent adverse event before birth as well as those who suffered an insult during birth. Furthermore this study did not separately analyse the one subset of cerebral palsy most convincingly associated with birth asphyxia and subsequent encephalopathy, namely athetoid / dyskinetic cerebral palsy.

The study also showed that almost 90% of survivors with a very low score did **not** have cerebral palsy and 80% of those **with** cerebral palsy had an Apgar score of 7 or more. This agrees well with an American study which showed that 80% of survivors with a score of 3 or less were entirely normal at school age.[127]

Virginia Apgar certainly drew attention to features which are important in assessing condition at birth but assigning scores to these features seems to have been much less helpful. The respiratory and heart rate scores are more important than the other items and the total score on its own is particularly uninformative. When one considers that each of the five components of the score is a separate ordinal variable it is perhaps not surprising that adding them together (a mathematically inappropriate manoeuvre for this level of measurement) is unhelpful.[174]

While it has long been assumed that a close relationship exists between the Apgar score and pH and umbilical blood gas status at birth, Sykes et al showed that this is not so.[177] Only 21% of babies with a 1-minute Apgar score of less than 7, and 19% of babies with a 5-minute score of less than 7 had an umbilical artery blood pH of less than 7·1. Conversely 73% with severe acidosis had a 1-minute Apgar score of 7 or more, while 86% had a 5-minute score of 7 or more.

In practice the Apgar score is usually recorded retrospectively and subjectively. For these reasons it may be highly unreliable. Many hospitals have never recorded this score and a number of others no longer do so. If it is your practice to record the Apgar score, a written description of all the characteristics used to assign the score must also be recorded as well as the details of any resuscitation.

	Apgar score		
Score	**0**	**1**	**2**
Colour	Pale/blue	Body pink, extremities blue	Pink
Heart rate	Absent	Less than 100	More than 100
Response to stimulation	Nil	Some movement	Cry
Muscle tone	Limp	Some flexion of extremities	Well flexed
Respiratory effort	Absent	Weak cry or hypoventilation	Good

Sarnat grading

In a baby who receives significant resuscitation at birth and who goes on to show signs of encephalopathy it is important to document the neurological state regularly over the first few days and not just at birth. The most useful system for this purpose is the Sarnat grading.[161] An assessment at 24 - 48 hours gives a much better indication of the long-term prognosis that any permutation of the 1, 5 and 10 minute Apgar score.[102]

Early fits (before 48 hours) are worrying, but signs of a moderate or severe encephalopathy at 24 - 48 hours correlate more closely with the long-term outcome two years and eight years later.[102, 155] It would seem much more useful to record the Sarnat grade at 48 hours in every term baby suspected of intrapartum 'asphyxia' than to record the Apgar score.

Early neonatal fits are not always due to intrapartum stress: neither is early neonatal encephalopathy, but intrapartum stress is certainly the commonest cause of early encephalopathy in the term baby, and the chance that the encephalopathy is related to intrapartum events is enhanced if there is other evidence of organ dysfunction.[165] The threshold for recognising mild (Sarnat Grade 1) encephalopathy probably varies in different centres, but most units can expect to encounter 2-3 babies with Grade 2 or Grade 3 encephalopathy per 1,000 births. Signs of encephalopathy need to be documented daily; better documentation of the duration of symptoms is likely to improve the prognostic power of the Sarnat grading system.

Sarnat grade			
Grade	**1**	**2**	**3**
Conscious level	Hyperalert	Lethargic or obtunded	Stuporous or comatose
Muscle tone	Normal	Mild hypotonia	Flaccid
Posture	Mild distal flexion	Strong distal flexion	Intermittent decerebration
Stretch reflexes	Overactive	Overactive	Decreased or absent
Moro reflex	Strong	Incomplete	Absent
Suck reflex	Normal	Weak or absent	Absent
Tonic neck reflex	Slight	Strong	Absent
Pupils	Dilated	Constricted	Poorly reactive
Gut motility	Normal	Increased	Variable
Seizures	Uncommon	Focal or multifocal	Mostly decerebrate

22 Preparing for a resuscitation

Objective

▶ **This chapter describes some of the preparation necessary before resuscitation. It involves your institution in making decisions about what kind of neonatal care it provides, identifying and training the right personnel and acquiring suitable equipment.**

You should personally familiarise yourself with local working practices and equipment. While preparing for an individual birth, you must anticipate the likely course of events, agree your role in the forthcoming resuscitation and know how to call for help. You must always be prepared for the possibility that the baby may need more resuscitation than you anticipated.

Advance preparation

Your institution, your employer, and you, should consider neonatal resuscitation in advance. Clear policies should be formulated in respect of the kind of resuscitations you are likely to face. Communication and transfer arrangements and pathways should be agreed with other providers if complex cases are to be referred on.

Different settings

To some extent, the need for resuscitation at birth can be predicted from antenatal and intrapartum risk factors. The pattern of care in the UK is to offer women different care settings, depending on the clinical situation and the mother's own preference. For instance a home birth with midwives in attendance might be considered for a multigravida with a normal pregnancy, whereas transfer before delivery to an obstetric unit with neonatal intensive care facilities would be advised for a woman in threatened preterm labour at 25 weeks. However, all professionals providing intrapartum care must remember that a baby can be born needing urgent resuscitation after an apparently normal pregnancy and delivery.

Arrangements for initiating resuscitation, calling for help and timely transfer of women in labour and babies after birth must be in place wherever babies are born.[202] Important details must be worked out in advance. For instance, in an emergency does the midwife conducting a birth at home dial 999 or call the local labour ward? Does she use a radio or a mobile telephone? Who will come to assist her: ambulance paramedics, a general practitioner, or an obstetric flying squad?

Training

Practitioners must be well trained. Theoretical and practical training such as that provided in courses run by the Resuscitation Council (UK), European Resuscitation Council or the American Heart Association in the USA, have been shown to be effective in providing a basic understanding and practical skills. Further mentored clinical experience will be required to achieve competence.

Equipment preparation and checking

Equipment must be prepared in advance [see Chapter 25] and you need to know how your equipment works and where it is kept. Equipment should also be checked regularly. However, when attending a delivery, check again, focussing on the items you are most likely to need for the case in hand. For preterm deliveries and when expecting an ill baby, check that a pulse oximeter is available. For all deliveries, make sure you have immediately available, the means to dry and cover the baby, open the airway, provide mask ventilation and call for help. Know where the equipment for more complex situations is kept.

Immediate preparation

When preparing for a specific case, you must think about the obstetric history, anticipate the likely course of the resuscitation, assemble the right team and check that you have the equipment prepared.

Obstetric history

In UK hospital practice, by the time a woman gives birth, an enormous amount of information is usually available about her, the pregnancy and the fetus. There are a large number of risk factors associated with a higher chance that the newborn will require active resuscitation. To list all these risk factors would be to write a textbook of obstetrics. In complex pregnancies, a perinatal plan is often made and recorded in the mother's obstetric notes. Always talk to the mother and midwifery and obstetric staff and review the notes when attending a delivery. When time is short, check for the limited number of very important risk factors which lead to a greatly increased risk that the baby will need resuscitation:

- Prematurity: Preterm babies have low drive, weak respiratory muscles and stiff lungs. They are also more susceptible to heat loss and have smaller glycogen reserves

- Multiple birth: There will be more than one baby to consider; the second and subsequent babies are likely to have more problems than the first

- Presence of thick meconium: Indicates possible problems with the fetus and can occasionally result in airway problems

Assemble the right team

Very few babies need resuscitation. However, there must always be one birth attendant available to look after the baby. This person must also be aware of the arrangements for summoning extra help. He or she should be capable of drying, warming and assessing the baby, opening the airway and providing mask ventilation.

Where a more complex situation is expected it may be helpful to have two or more people available for the baby. A number of tasks may need to be undertaken and appropriately coordinated in a relatively short timescale. In addition to simple management of the airway these might include fitting a pulse oximeter probe, intubation, obtaining vascular access and finding and mixing drugs.

Where a significantly preterm baby is expected, especially one of 30 weeks gestation or less, a senior paediatrician with extensive experience in dealing with preterm babies should be present at the delivery to supervise the resuscitation stabilisation and transfer to the neonatal unit.

Parents

Talk to the mother and her birth partner. Introduce yourself and the members of your team and explain briefly what you are going to do for the baby, what they are likely to see and that you will talk to them again afterwards.

Summary

▷ **Successful resuscitation is dependent on forward planning. As far as possible, babies should be born in a setting where their needs for resuscitation and further care can be met. Birth attendants involved in newborn resuscitation should be adequately trained. The right equipment must be available and working. Before an individual delivery, the likely course of events should be anticipated and an appropriate team should be assembled. They should check equipment and decide on team roles before the delivery.**

23 A cautionary note

> ### 'When we all think alike, no one is thinking'
>
> Lipmann W. Public Opinion. Harcourt Brace & Co. 1922

This manual is a consensus statement and one should always be sceptical of such statements. Just because everyone agrees you should do something a particular way does not mean that that really is the best way to do it. We would do well to remember the words of Sir Thomas Allbutt, *"our path is cumbered with guesses, presumptions and conjectures, the untimely and sterile fruitage of minds which cannot bear to wait for the facts, and are ready to forget that the use of hypothesis lies not in the display of ingenuity but in the labour of verification"*.

There are many controversies in the field of neonatal resuscitation and little strong experimental evidence is currently available to resolve them. Publication of an opinion, even in a highly reputable journal, does not mean that that opinion is correct. In 1951 a leading article in the Lancet entitled Anoxia in the Newborn confidently stated that '*any method of attempting pulmonary expansion by blowing gases into the trachea under pressure must be condemned'.*[44] We now know that this is not only safe, but in certain circumstances it is a highly desirable practice.

In the 1960s respiratory stimulants were commonly used but we now know them to be both ineffective and potentially dangerous. Even in the 21st century many experts have strongly recommended that the nose and mouth of the baby should be aspirated before the shoulders were delivered in labours complicated by meconium stained liquor. This practice has been recommended since the 1970s and large amounts of money have presumably changed hands in court cases based on whether this advice was or was not followed. However, since 2004 we know from a large multi-centre randomised controlled study that such intrapartum suctioning is not effective in preventing meconium aspiration syndrome.[193] Many other examples exist. Future work will hopefully resolve some of these controversies but others will certainly arise to take their place.

Much of the physiological evidence on which the strategies of neonatal resuscitation are based relates to sudden total asphyxia. In real life intermittent partial asphyxia of varying severity, frequency and duration, with or without accompanying ischaemia, is the more common pattern of intrapartum insult that the fetus has to face. The physiological response to this pattern of stresses is less well explored and may be subtly different. Furthermore, the response of a chronically stressed baby whose intrauterine growth has been compromised may well be different to that of a well grown baby facing significant problems for the first time. Heart rate responses to stress in labour differ between male and female babies. It is also likely that the quality and nature of any fetal responses will vary with varying degrees of fetal maturity.

While the current enthusiasm for detailed protocols continues it should be remembered that a protocol is only as good as the experimental evidence on which it is based. The advice in this manual constitutes a *guide* to resuscitation at birth, not a protocol. It represents the collective opinion of many with extensive personal experience of performing neonatal resuscitation as well as teaching the subject. The advice given does not define the only way that resuscitation at birth should be performed. We merely suggest that it is an accepted view of how resuscitation at birth can be carried out both safely and effectively.

Controversies

> ## 'In God we trust; all others must bring data'
>
> W Edwards Deming

Introduction

When considering the practicalities of newborn resuscitation one encounters a number of controversial areas. Most of these are capable of generating an amount of heated argument quite out of proportion to their importance. Nevertheless these controversies still cause distress, confusion and debate and some controversies are of greater potential importance. This chapter will attempt to set out some of the evidence on either side of the various debates and put the arguments in context.

When should the umbilical cord be clamped?

This question has been asked in various forms for at least 200 years and the issue is now being debated once again. So-called 'active management of the third stage of labour' was introduced in the 1970s primarily to address the problem of post-partum haemorrhage. Such active management involves giving an intramuscular injection of syntometrine to the mother immediately after emergence of the baby, with the cord usually being clamped before the injection was given. Little thought appears to have been given to any effect on the baby.

There have been a number of studies comparing 'early' versus so-called 'delayed' clamping of the cord. The definition of what constitutes 'early' clamping varies between 'immediate', less than 20 seconds, less than 1 minute and in the early literature less than 5 minutes. Definition of late clamping has been similarly variable.

Clamping of the cord before the baby has taken a breath is associated with a drop in heart rate that is not seen if clamping occurs after the first breath.[22] When viewed on video-radiography, a decrease in heart size for three or four cardiac cycles is seen if clamping occurs before the first breath.[140] One suggested reason for this is that the increased cardiac output necessary to begin filling the pulmonary circulation, which normally occurs with the first few breaths, is easily replenished from the placenta via the umbilical circulation if the cord is unclamped. If this is the correct explanation then clearly this rapid replenishment cannot occur if breathing does not start until after the cord is clamped. Venous return to the heart is then temporarily inadequate for a few beats until blood begins to return from the lungs into the left atrium. However, studies of placental transfusion rate and uterine contraction failed to show any clear relationship between infant blood volume in the first hour of life and timing of cord clamping in relation to establishment of regular respiration.[210]

How the total volume of blood in the conceptus is distributed between the placenta and the baby can change during labour and at delivery. Furthermore, pressure on the cord, such as might occlude the soft-walled umbilical vein but fail to occlude the muscular-walled umbilical arteries, has been held responsible for neonatal hypovolaemia sufficient to cause shock.[194] There are also concerns that a similar process whereby pressure on the fetal thorax in the birth canal during obstructed labour, for example in shoulder dystocia, may transfer a significant volume of blood from the compressed fetus to the placenta. If the cord is then clamped and cut before the compression is relieved by the birth of the baby, then this blood cannot return from the placenta, which might leave the baby seriously hypovolaemic.[117]

In term babies iron status in infancy is certainly improved by later clamping at birth, presumably because it allows a greater placental transfusion to the baby after delivery. An increase in clinical jaundice and use of phototherapy has been reported in various studies but this is perhaps less worrying than it first appears given that the criteria for the use of phototherapy were neither defined nor controlled and more invasive treatment of jaundice was apparently not required.

In preterm infants the observed benefits of later clamping are greater stability in immediate postnatal transition, more stable blood pressure, reduced use of pressor agents and a reduced perceived necessity for early or later transfusion.[3, 11, 116, 147] Also, waiting before clamping the cord might conceivably increase the passage of stem cells to the baby.[186] Worries about increased jaundice, unintentional hypothermia, increased need for exchange transfusion for hyperbilirubinaemia (or polycythaemia), or increased respiratory distress have not been confirmed.[147]

Unfortunately babies apparently needing significant resuscitation were excluded from all these studies so it is not possible to say with any certainty whether later cord clamping is appropriate under those circumstances. Furthermore, the physiological animal studies described in chapter 5 were all done with the umbilical cord occluded at the onset of asphyxia and later divided. Any effect of re-establishment of the feto-placental circulation in the treatment of asphyxia was therefore not explored.

It should perhaps be remembered that, although it may be more *convenient* to transfer the baby to a resuscitaire to provide resuscitation such transfer is not an essential feature of resuscitation itself. Indeed, if the placenta has not separated from the uterine wall, it may even be advantageous to the baby to start resuscitation without clamping or cutting the cord.[43]

Where are we now?

In 2007 The World Health Organisation published recommendations for the prevention of postpartum haemorrhage, which state: *"Because of the benefits to the baby, the cord should not be clamped earlier than is necessary for applying cord traction in the active management of the third stage of labour. [weak recommendation, low quality evidence]. For the sake of clarity, it is estimated that this will normally take around 3 minutes. Early clamping may be required if the baby is asphyxiated and requires immediate resuscitation."* [207]

In 2009 the Royal College of Obstetricians and Gynaecologists published a Scientific Advisory Committee opinion entitled 'Clamping of the umbilical cord and placental transfusion'.[158] They acknowledge that *"for decades immediate cord clamping has been bundled into the package of care known as 'active management' and the potential consequences either ignored or forgotten"*. They also strongly support further investigation of this issue by means of large randomised controlled trials.

In 2010 the International Liaison Committee on Resuscitation (ILCOR) considered the published evidence and issued the following recommendation: *"Delay in umbilical cord clamping for at least 1 minute is recommended for newborn infants not requiring resuscitation. There is insufficient evidence to support or refute a recommendation to delay cord clamping in babies requiring resuscitation."* [142, 209] In the preamble to this recommendation they stated *"There are limited data on the hazards or benefits of delayed cord clamping in the non-vigorous infant"*.

What should drive clamping of the cord? Should it wait until the baby takes a spontaneous breath, or until cord pulsation has ceased, or should it wait a specific length of time: if this last, then what length of time is appropriate and might that time differ following delivery by section or if blood in the cord was 'milked' towards the baby before clamping? Is this pause affected by the timing, dose or route of administration of uterotonics? Should this pause also occur if the baby has no detectable heart rate at delivery or should one consider milking the cord before clamping in this situation? Should the cord be clamped before providing positive pressure ventilation? Should the same instructions apply to all babies – including both those apparently needing resuscitation and those born very preterm?

Randomised controlled trials are urgently needed to address questions such as these and such trials should involve all babies, including those apparently needing resuscitation and the very preterm. Perinatal

consequences of early and later clamping to both the mother and the baby need to be evaluated in these trials and neuro-developmental outcomes should also be compared, particularly in relation to preterm babies.

Use of CPAP and/or PEEP at birth

When attending the delivery of preterm infants, one is more commonly involved in stabilisation of a fragile infant rather than resuscitation of a nearly dead one. In the absence of good evidence to act differently one might reasonably suppose that gentle support of spontaneous respiration, perhaps with CPAP alone, rather than immediate intubation, might have advantages. Certainly changes in strategy along these lines have apparently resulted in reduced intubation and ventilation rates of babies less than 1000g with no apparent increase in morbidity – at least in the dubious context of a prospective study with historic controls.[108]

Continuous positive airway pressure or CPAP has been around since the 1950s but has attracted renewed interest in the past ten years. A randomised controlled trial in preterm lambs has shown that the group receiving CPAP had higher lung volumes and less histological evidence of inflammation than a comparison group who were ventilated from birth.[85]

Of course, early application of CPAP with the intention of avoiding intubation will deprive the baby of the advantages of early vs. later administration of surfactant supplementation. However, perhaps the early application of CPAP, rather than more aggressive ventilation at delivery (which is usually given without positive end expiratory pressure [PEEP]), might avoid accelerated destruction of any endogenous surfactant which might be present.[146]

No-one would ventilate a baby on the neonatal unit without PEEP because in this situation PEEP prevents the infant's lung from completely deflating during expiration and thus obviates any need for re-aeration from scratch with each new inspiration. In other words it helps to preserve the functional reserve capacity of the lung. Use of PEEP from the outset in the ventilation of newborn animals has been shown to reduce the amount of lung inflammation and to preserve surfactant function in preterm animal models.[146]

CPAP and PEEP can be delivered by modern T-piece systems during resuscitation without any need for dedicated CPAP drivers - see Chapter 25, Fig 15.1.

Sodium bicarbonate

This manual recommends that drugs should only be used in those very rare situations where the heart rate has not responded to adequate lung aeration, ventilation and well performed chest compression. Some, however, have significant reservations about using bicarbonate.[70] On closer inspection these reservations relate to the practice of rapidly correcting acidosis following resuscitation or infusion of bicarbonate routinely during resuscitation - reservations which are reasonable. However, it does not follow that bicarbonate should not be used at all.

Some of the early work on animals examined the effect of injecting either respiratory stimulants or base intravenously (in this case tris-hydroxymethyl-aminomethane or THAM, an organic base) in asphyxiated fetal monkeys when they were known to have taken their last gasp and thus known to be in terminal apnoea.[35] The injection of the respiratory stimulants lobeline or nikethamide resulted in a fall in blood pressure whereas the injection of THAM (0·5% molar solution with 3·5% dextrose - pH adjusted to 8·85) caused a rise in both heart rate and blood pressure and the recurrence of gasping allowing the monkeys to be successfully resuscitated using positive pressure ventilation. This is why this text would like to be able to recommend that bicarbonate or THAM be considered if adequate lung aeration, ventilation and chest compression achieve no increase in heart rate.

Unfortunately, no-one thought to investigate the effect of adrenaline in the experiment described in the previous paragraph. Animal data shows that the binding of adrenaline to its receptors in the myocardium is significantly impaired by lactic acidosis and recent work on human lymphocyte beta-adrenergic receptors supports this view.[121] Whether this is also true of the more important alpha receptors is unknown.

Intratracheal adrenaline

In order to overcome some of the delay associated with intravenous administration of adrenaline at newborn resuscitation it has been suggested that adrenaline can be effective when given down the tracheal tube into the lungs.[106] Few of the animal studies of this technique have been done in newborn animals whose lungs have just been aerated. It appears to be effective in adult (human) resuscitation provided a dose of at least 2 mg of adrenaline is given.[149] However, recent work in newborn piglets suggests that while doses given intravenously had measurable effects on carotid blood pressure, similar doses given via the tracheal tube had no measurable effect.[94]

Evidence from one case series showed response was more common after intravenous adrenaline than after a similar dose of tracheal adrenaline.[12] This is consistent with evidence extrapolated from neonatal animal models indicating that higher doses (50 - 100 microgram/kg) of tracheal adrenaline may be required to achieve the increased blood adrenaline concentrations and haemodynamic responses seen after intravenous administration.[31, 84] Although it has been widely assumed that adrenaline can be administered faster by the tracheal route, no clinical trials have evaluated this hypothesis. Whether effective or not, if you want to give tracheal adrenaline then a tracheal tube needs to be in place.

Naloxone and maternal opiate abuse

Many guidelines on resuscitation at birth warn against giving naloxone to the baby of an opiate abusing mother for fear of inducing fits.[142, 209] As justification for this statement all quote the same single case report of fits in a newborn baby apparently from this cause.[58] No further reports have been published or reported on the 'yellow card' scheme in the 21 years since this report and naloxone does not cause adult opiate abusers to fit if given after an opiate overdose. It is probable that the infant of a mother who has been regularly abusing opiates in pregnancy is less likely to have respiratory depression from maternal opiates given in labour than an infant whose mother had not used opiates before.

Intraosseous access

There is no evidence for the effectiveness or otherwise of intraosseous infusion of drugs in resuscitation at birth. Recent data suggest that the intraosseous route can be effective in the resuscitation of preterm and full term infants in the intensive care unit when alternative venous access proves impossible to establish.[46] However, it is difficult to justify the insertion of such a device into the bone of a newborn baby when umbilical venous catheterisation so easily provides central venous access of known efficacy. The technique should perhaps be reserved for those extremely rare occasions when a baby requiring resuscitation at birth also has a problem, such as exomphalos, which makes umbilical venous catheterisation more difficult.

When to offer increased oxygen?

If damaging hyperoxia could be avoided, might concentrations of inhaled oxygen greater than 21% result in faster and more complete resolution of cellular asphyxia? Only if the concentration of inspired oxygen is the limiting factor to the speed of the processes involved – and there is little evidence to support this.

There is no clear, evidence-based, recommendation that can be given as to when to offer an increased concentration of oxygen during resuscitation other than when a baby remains cyanosed despite effective ventilation. However the failure of a baby's heart rate to respond to apparently effective ventilation (confirmed by chest movement) is a reasonable indication that the situation may require an extended resuscitation and at this point the issue of whether higher concentrations of oxygen might prove helpful should be *considered* (and may, quite reasonably, be rejected) – though the immediate *practical* response should be to proceed to chest compressions.

In the absence of a heart rate response to lung aeration, establishment of a circulation to deliver oxygenated blood to the heart and other organs can only be achieved by chest compressions with ventilation. The situation is unlikely to be materially influenced by an increase in the inspired oxygen concentration. However, once the heart rate has responded, if the baby remains cyanosed then an increase in oxygen concentration might again be considered. Whenever increased oxygen is offered the dosage should ideally be monitored by pulse oximetry.

25 Equipment: a discussion

Introduction

In essence, the requirements for neonatal resuscitation are those described by Barrie in the influential article he published in the Lancet in 1963 when the techniques now in universal use were first being established.[14]

Since that time the tracheal tube has been replaced as an "essential requirement" by the modern silicone mask, and the T-piece has been developed. It has also been recognised that air is as effective as 100% oxygen and yet safer.[148, 152] A stethoscope and a clock can be helpful. Overhead radiant heat is useful, but it is no substitute for minimising evaporative heat loss by drying the baby and wrapping it in warm, dry towels to avoid draughts. Few babies should need to remain on the resuscitation trolley for more than ten minutes after birth. A list of suggested equipment can be found on the Resuscitation Council (UK) website.

Working surface

This should be warm, flat, firm and well lit.

Masks

The ideal facemask is a round, soft silicone mask with an easily deformable surface which, when placed against the baby's face, will mould around the facial contours and form a good air-tight seal as described by Palme et al in 1985.[137] Size 0/1 is best for most babies, but size 00 will be required for very small babies. An appropriately sized anatomical face mask with similar soft, easily deformable sealing surface, is also suitable [see fig 8.5 in Chap 8].

T-pieces

T-piece devices are designed to be attached to pressurised gas supplies via systems which allow one to regulate both the flow of gas through the T-piece and the maximum pressure that can be delivered. This maximum pressure is controlled by an adjustable pressure blow-off valve and most systems also have a back-up safety blow-off valve.

If the pressure blow-off valve is set to deliver a specific pressure it should be remembered that if the flow is subsequently changed then the blow-off pressure will also change because the blow-off valves are flow-dependent.

> ### T-PIECES SHOULD NEVER BE CONNECTED DIRECTLY TO WALL GAS SUPPLIES

T-piece systems have a number of advantages over self-inflating bags. They can provide PEEP or CPAP which can be adjusted by a screw device on the T-piece itself. As both the flow and the peak pressure are adjustable and regulated, T-pieces also provide a more constant pressure delivery than bag-valve systems. Provision of timed inflation breaths or ventilations is also more accurate. However, they can only be used if a pressurised gas supply is available.

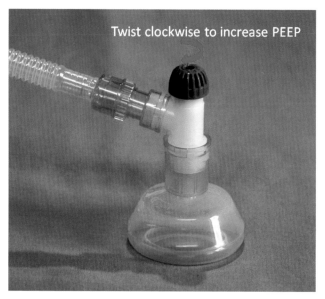

Fig 25.1 T-piece with adjustable CPAP/PEEP

Self-inflating bags

Self-inflating bags are useful for providing gas under pressure when a compressed gas supply is not available. Bags of about 500 ml are more appropriate than smaller volume bags for resuscitation of term babies at birth.[50]

Only use a bag which also incorporates a pressure limiting device and be aware that on some makes of self-inflating bag it is possible to 'lock' the blow-off valve closed - this leaves the valve unable to blow-off until it has been 'unlocked'. Always test the bag's blow-off valve before using it (Figure 25.2). Seal the outlet to the baby and squeeze the bag. You should hear the blow-off valve working as the pressure rises, if you do not hear this, check the valve mechanism.

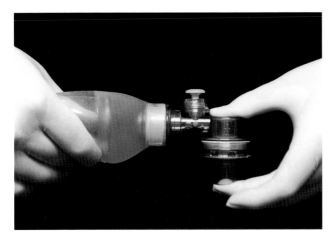

Fig 25.2 Testing the blow-off valve

Aim to produce a pressure of about 30 cm water and then sustain it at that level for 2 - 3 seconds for each of the first five breaths. Make a good seal with the mask on the baby's face and then squeeze the bag slowly until the valve begins to open, you then know you have reached the appropriate pressure. Continue squeezing hard enough to keep the valve blowing as long as possible. Do not squeeze the bag very rapidly as this risks producing rapid gas flow sufficient to override the blow-off valve and delivery of higher pressures to the baby than you would wish.[51]

> **ALWAYS TEST THE BLOW-OFF VALVE BEFORE USING A BAG**

Giving oxygen with bags

Most self-inflating bags come with some form of detachable oxygen reservoir. The instructions that come with these bags often suggest that only 40% oxygen is delivered if oxygen is connected direct to the bag without a reservoir in place. In fact this is not so and at least some of these bags will deliver anything from 30% to 70% oxygen in this situation, depending on the flow rate used.[183]

Gas

It is best to start resuscitation with air. Additional oxygen is very rarely needed. If it is thought to be necessary it should be given via an air/oxygen blender and the effect monitored using pulse oximetry. All maternity units in the UK will have piped oxygen and many will also have piped air. Where piped air is not available, a supply of compressed air in a cylinder can nearly always be supplied. Gas flows of about 6 litre min[-1] may be necessary during facemask resuscitation in order to compensate for the larger dead-space, but a lower flow may be sufficient when resuscitating an intubated baby - in this situation flows much in excess of 4 litre min[-1] can produce an abrupt rise in airway pressure that might be traumatic.

Pulse oximetry

Pulse oximetry gives a quick and relatively accurate display of both heart rate and oxygen saturation which can be easily seen by all involved in the resuscitation. This is particularly useful when stabilising significantly preterm babies or when tempted to give additional oxygen to any baby.

The pulse oximeter probe should ideally be fitted to the right hand or wrist, this will give pre-ductal oxygen saturation values. However, fitting the probe takes time and the machine also needs to boot-up before it can start to give information. With practice, reliable data can be obtained within about 90 seconds of delivery.[130]

Set the data acquisition sensitivity to maximum and the data averaging time to the shortest available (~2 seconds). Once the oximeter is switched on, a reading can be obtained a few seconds faster if the probe is first attached to the baby and only then connected to the machine.[130] Once the heart rate is displayed it is likely that this will be more accurate than other commonly used methods of assessing heart rate.

Stethoscopes

Heart rate: Though it is often possible to assess the heart rate of a baby by feeling either for a pulse in the umbilical cord stump or by observing or feeling the pulsation of the ventricle against the chest wall, neither of these methods is infallible. Listening for a heart rate with a stethoscope is much more reliable. If a stethoscope is used then it is important to get one with a chest piece small enough to use on a small baby. However, a stethoscope does not provide a reliable way of checking whether air is entering the lung because the sound of air entering the stomach is all too easily transmitted into the chest. A stethoscope can, however, be useful in detecting cardiac displacement and in determining whether air entry is equal on both sides of the chest.

Displaced tracheal tube: Listening with a stethoscope at the mouth may help to determine whether a tube is in fact in the oesophagus. If there is a very audible leak when you apply positive pressure then it is likely to be in the oesophagus.

Suction

Most modern resuscitation trolleys provide facilities for mechanical suction but this is only rarely needed at birth. If suction is necessary then it will be to remove thick particulate matter from the oropharynx or the airway and a relatively large bore suction catheter will be needed. Any suction catheter that is thinner than 12 or 14 French gauge is unlikely to be useful for this purpose. An adaptor made to fit the 15 mm standard anaesthetic connection on the end of the tracheal tube will allow suction directly via the tracheal tube and this is the most effective method of clearing the trachea of significant debris [see illustration on page 50].

Laryngoscopes

An infant size laryngoscope blade is essential and a lightweight handle is an advantage. A straight blade with the light emerging fairly near the tip is almost certainly the best. We recommend the Oxford blade, with a useful if disconcertingly large tongue guard, as being best for beginners even with small babies. The smallest size Wisconsin blade is useful for babies less than 1000g. The Robertshaw style of blade is probably the best of the neonatal blades without a tongue guard. Laryngoscope blades should be autoclavable or even for single-patient use only.

Tracheal tubes

Uncuffed tracheal tubes made to Magill's basic design are probably the best all-purpose tubes for resuscitation and for prolonged oral or nasal intubation in the newborn.

Laryngeal mask airways

The laryngeal mask airway (LMA) is a small elliptical mask with an inflatable rim connected to an airway tube. The mask is inserted orally using the operator's index finger and guided along the hard palate over the tongue to the hypopharynx. Once inserted, the rim is inflated and the mask sits with its lumen facing the laryngeal opening while the rim conforms to the contours of the hypopharynx and occludes the oesophagus with a low-pressure seal. The airway tube includes an adaptor that is attached to a positive pressure device. In babies of 2000g or more they can be very helpful in achieving airway control especially if face mask inflation or intubation is problematic.[139] There is limited evidence in smaller babies but case reports suggest that LMAs can be used successfully in this group.

Carbon dioxide detection

Studies suggest that detection of exhaled CO_2 confirms tracheal intubation in neonates with cardiac output more rapidly and accurately than clinical assessment alone.[77, 151, 154] There is no comparative information to allow recommendation of any one method for detection of exhaled CO_2 in the neonatal population.

Colorimetric methods for detecting CO_2 are commonly used to determine whether a tube is placed in the airway. Carbon dioxide is detected by a pH sensitive chemical indicator enclosed in a plastic housing and exposed to the gas stream returning from the patient. If sufficient CO_2 is detected in the gas stream then the colour changes from purple to yellow before returning to purple as the CO_2 concentration falls. Colorimetric detectors are available for babies weighing more than 1000g. However, it is possible to use them in smaller babies.[57] In babies weighing less than 750g there may not be sufficient chest recoil and, if the tracheal tube is thought to be in place, one or two chest compressions may be required to provide sufficient volume of exhaled breath to register on the device.

Though capable of a very quick response,[9] there are some limitations to the use of these devices. Liquids spilt on the detector such as adrenaline, surfactant or gastric contents can cause a change to yellow thus falsely suggesting that the tube is correctly placed. Also one can be misled about a correctly placed tube if the cardiac output is so low as to fail to deliver sufficient CO_2 to the baby's lungs.[9, 78]

Drugs

The drugs required when dealing with a sudden cardio-respiratory arrest in adult life are not the same as those used in the newborn period. The only drugs used are adrenaline (1:10,000), sodium bicarbonate (8·4% which ideally should be diluted 1:1 before administration, or 4·2%) - an alternative base would be Tris-hydroxymethyl-aminomethane [THAM], dextrose (5% or 10%), and some volume expander (such as 0·9% saline).

Other drugs can be asked for if they are needed. Their routine presence on the resuscitation trolley only causes unnecessary confusion.

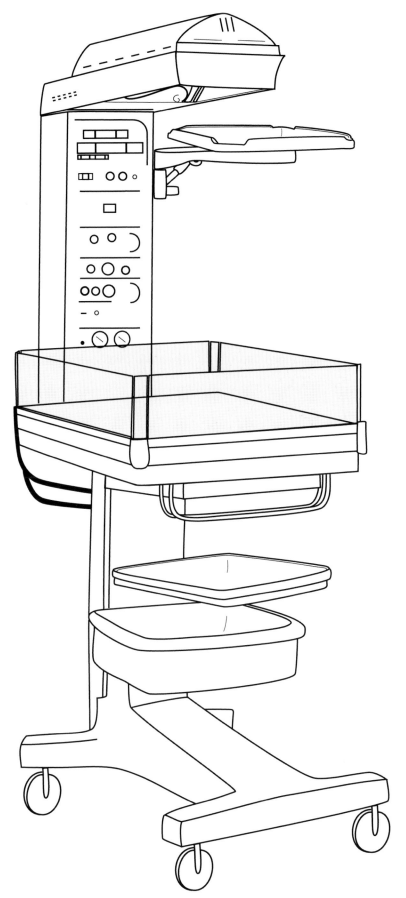

Overhead heater & light

Stop clock

Pulse oximeter on shelf

Equipment on top of resuscitaire
Towels
Stethoscope
T connector and tubing
Face masks (sizes 0/1 and 00)
Scissors
Yankauer sucker

Equipment below working surface
Plastic bag for preterm infants
Laryngoscopes with Oxford infant blade
Spare laryngoscope and Wisconsin blade
Oropharyngeal airways sizes 00 and 000
Three tracheal tubes of each size (2.5, 3.0 & 3.5)
Three packs of cord scissors & umbilical clamp
Six 21 gauge (green) needles
Six 25 gauge (orange) needles
Roll of ½ inch adhesive tape

Emergency box
One pair Magill's forceps
Two umbilical venous catheters
One umbilical catheterisation pack
Two ampoules of adrenaline 1 in 10,000
Two ampoules of sodium bicarbonate
10% dextrose
Five ampoules of 0.9% saline (10 ml)
Five syringes (10 ml)
Five needles (21 G)
One bag of Hartmann's (500 ml)
One three-way tap
Two 22 gauge butterfly needles
Two black silk sutures
Two scalpel blades
Two sterile heparinised syringes (2 ml)

References

1. Adamsons K Jr, Behrman R, Dawes GS, *et al.* Resuscitation by positive pressure ventilation and Tris-hydroxymethyl-aminomethane in rhesus monkeys asphyxiated at birth. *J Pediatr* 1964; **65**: 807-18.

2. Akerren Y, Furstenberg N. Gastrointestinal administration of oxygen in the treatment of asphyxia in the newborn. *J Obstet Gynaecol Br Emp* 1950; **57**: 705-13.

3. Aladangady N, McHugh S, Aitchison TC *et al.* Infants' blood volume in a controlled trial of placental transfusion at preterm delivery. *Pediatrics* 2006; **117**: 93-8.

4. Allwood AC, Madar RJ, Baumer JH, *et al.* Changes in resuscitation practice at birth. *Arch Dis Child Fetal Neonatal Ed* 2003; **88**: F375-9.

5. American Thoracic Society / European Respiratory Society. Respiratory mechanics in infants: physiologic evaluation in health and disease. *Amer Rev Respir Dis* 1993; **147**: 474-96.

6. Apgar V. A proposal for a new method of evaluation of the newborn infant. *Anesth Analg (Clev)* 1953; **32**: 260-7.

7. Apgar V, James LS. Further observations on the Newborn Scoring System. *Amer J Dis Child* 1962; **104**: 419-28.

8. Armstrong L, Stenson B. The effect of delayed sampling on umbilical cord arterial and venous lactate and blood gases in clamped and unclamped vessels. *Arch Dis Child Fetal Neonatal Ed* 2006; **91**: F342-5

9. Aziz HF, Martin JB, Moore JJ. The pediatric disposable end-tidal carbon dioxide detector role in endotracheal intubation in newborns. *J Perinatol* 1999; **19**: 110-3.

10. Azzopardi DV, Strohm B, Edwards AD *et al.* Moderate hypothermia to treat perinatal asphyxial encephalopathy. *New Engl J Med* 2009; **361**: 1349-58.

11. Baenziger O, Stolkin F, Keel M *et al.* The influence of the timing of cord clamping on postnatal cerebral oxygenation in preterm neonates: a randomized, controlled trial. *Pediatrics* 2007; **119**: 455-9.

12. Barber CA, Wyckoff MH. Use and efficacy of endotracheal versus intravenous epinephrine during neonatal cardiopulmonary resuscitation in the delivery room. *Pediatrics* 2006; **118**: 1028–34.

13. Barrie H, Cottom DG, Wilson BDR. Respiratory stimulants in the newborn. *Lancet* 1962; **ii**: 742-6.

14. Barrie H. Resuscitation of the newborn. *Lancet* 1963; **i**: 650-5.

15. Benfield DG, Flaksman RJ, Lin T-H, *et al.* Teaching intubation skills using newly deceased infants *JAMA* 1991; **265**: 2360-3.

16. Bennett S, Finer NN, Rich W, Vaucher Y. A comparison of three neonatal resuscitation devices. *Resuscitation* 2005; **67**: 113-8.

17. Birch S, Rhodes H, Wylie P. Laryngeal damage from intubation (case report). *Br Med J* 1999; **318**: 614.

18. Björklund LJ, Ingimarsson J, Curstedt T, *et al.* Manual ventilation with a few large breaths at birth compromises the therapeutic effect of subsequent surfactant. *Pediatr Res* 1997; **42**: 348-55.

19. Blaikley LB, Gibberd GF. Asphyxia neonatorum: its treatment by tracheal intubation.. *Lancet* 1935; **i**: 736-9.

20. Bland RD. Lung liquid clearance before and after birth. *Semin Perinatol* 1988; **12**: 124-33.

21. Boon AW, Milner AD, Hopkin IE. Physiological responses of the newborn infant to resuscitation. *Arch Dis Child* 1979; **54**: 492-8.

22. Brady JP, James LS, Baker MA. Heart rate changes in the fetus and newborn infant during labor, delivery and the immediate neonatal period. *Am J Obstet Gynecol* 1962; **84**: 1-12.

23. Brattebø G, Wisborg T, Solheim K, Oyen N. Public opinion on different approaches to teaching intubation techniques. *Br Med J* 1993; **307**: 1256-7.

24. British Association of Perinatal Medicine. Position statement on therapeutic cooling for neonatal encephalopathy. July 2010. www.bapm.org.uk/

25. Cabal LA, Devaskar U, Siassi B, *et al.* Cardiogenic shock associated with perinatal asphyxia in preterm infants. *J Pediatr* 1980; **96**: 705-10.

26. Chamberlain R, Chamberlain G, Howlett B, Claireaux A. The first breath. Chapter 4 (p 89-117) in British Births 1970. Volume 1: The first week of life. Heinemann, London 1970.

27. Chan LC, Hey E. Can all neonatal resuscitation be managed by nurse practitioners? *Arch Dis Child Fetal Neonatal Ed* 2006; **91**: F52-5.

28. Cooper EA, Smith H, Pask EA. On the efficiency of intragastric oxygen. *Anaesthesia* 1960; **15**: 211-28.

29. Cordey R, Chiolero R, Miller J Jr. Resuscitation of neonates by hypothermia: report of 20 cases with acid-base determination on 10 cases and longterm development of 33 cases. *Resuscitation* 1973; **2**: 169-87.

30. Coxon RV. The effect of intragastric oxygen on the oxygenation of arterial and portal blood in hypoxic animals. *Lancet* 1960; **i**: 1315-7.

31. Crespo SG, Schoffstall JM, Fuhs LR, Spivey WH. Comparison of two doses of endotracheal epinephrine in a cardiac arrest model. *Ann Emerg Med* 1991; **20**: 230–4.

32. Cross KW, Dawes GS, Hyman A, Mott JC. Hyperbaric oxygen and intermittent positive pressure ventilation in resuscitation of asphyxiated newborn rabbits. *Lancet* 1964; **ii**: 560-2.

33. Cross KW. Resuscitation of the asphyxiated infant. *Brit Med Bull* 1966; **22**: 73-8.

34. Dahm LS, James LS. Newborn temperature and calculated heat loss in the delivery room. *Pediatrics* 1972; **49**: 504-13.

35. Daniel SS, Dawes GS, James LS, Ross BB. Analeptics and resuscitation of asphyxiated monkeys. *Br Med J* 1966; **ii**: 562-3.

36. David R. Closed chest cardiac massage in the newborn infant. *Pediatrics* 1988; **81**: 552-4.

37. Dawes G. Fetal and neonatal physiology. Year Book Publisher, Chicago, 1968; Chapter 12: 141-59.

38. Dawson JA, Kamlin COF, Vento M, *et al.* Defining the reference range for oxygen saturation for infants after birth. Pediatrics. 2010; 125:e1340-7.

39. Dawson JA, Kamlin COF, Wong C *et al.* Changes in heart rate in the first minutes after birth. *Arch Dis Child Fetal Neonatal Ed* 2010; **95**: F177-81.

40. Department of Health. National Service Framework for Children, Young People and Maternity Services. Standard 11: Maternity Services. Department of Health 2004.

41. Dimond B. The Legal Aspects of Midwifery. Books for Midwives Press, Cheshire, 1994.

42. Ditchburn RK, Hull D, Segall MM. Oxygen uptake during and after positive-pressure ventilation for the resuscitation of asphyxiated newborn infants. *Lancet* 1966; **ii**: 1096-9.

43. Dunn PM. Postnatal placental respiration. *Dev Med Child Neurol* 1966; **8**: 607-8.

44. Editorial. Anoxia in the newborn. *Lancet* 1951; **ii**: 821-2.

45. Edwards AD, Brocklehurst P, Gunn AJ *et al.* Neurological outcomes at 18 months of age after moderate hypothermia for perinatal hypoxic ischaemic encephalopathy: synthesis and meta-analysis of trial data. *Br Med J* 2010; **340**: c363 doi: 10.1136/bmj.c363.

46. Ellemunter H, Simma B, Trawöger R, Maurer H. Intraosseous lines in preterm and full term neonates. *Arch Dis Child Fetal Neonatal Ed* 1999; **80**: F74-5.

47. Eve FC. Actuation of the inert diaphragm by a gravity method. *Lancet* 1932; **ii**: 995-7.

48. Eve FC. Complacency in resuscitation of the drowned. *Br Med J* 1943; **i**: 535-7.

49. Falciglia HS, Henderschott C, Potter P, Helmchen R. Does De Lee suction at the perineum prevent meconium aspiration syndrome. *Amer J Obstet Gynecol* 1992; **167**: 1243-9.

50. Field D, Milner AD, Hopkin IE. Efficiency of manual resuscitators at birth. *Arch Dis Child* 1986; **61**: 300-2.

51. Finer NN, Barrington KJ, al-Fadley F, Peters KL. Limitations of self-inflating resuscitators. *Pediatrics* 1986; **77**: 417-20.

52. Finer NN, Rich W, Craft A, Henderson C. Comparison of methods of bag and mask ventilation for neonatal resuscitation. *Resuscitation* 2001; **49**: 299-305.

53. Flagg PJ. The treatment of asphyxia in the newborn. *JAMA* 1928; **91**: 788-91.

54. Gallagher B, Neligan G. Resuscitation of the stillborn infant. *Br Med J* 1962; **i**: 400.

55. Galos G, Surks S. Cardiorespiratory arrest in the newborn treated by cardiac massage. A report of two cases. *Am J Obstet Gynecol* 1957; **74**: 1108-11.

56. Gandy GM, Adamsons K, Cunningham N, *et al*. Thermal environment and acid-base homeostasis in human infants during the first few hours of life. *J Clin Invest* 1964; **43**: 751-8.

57. Garey DM, Rich W, Heldt G *et al*. Tidal volume threshold for colorimetric carbon dioxide detectors available for use in neonates. *Pediatrics* 2008; **121**: e1524-7

58. Gibbs J, Newson T, Williams J, Davidson DC. Naloxone hazard in infant of opioid abuser. *Lancet* 1989; **ii**: 159-60.

59. Gluck L, Kulovich MV, Eidelman AI, *et al*. Biochemical development of surface activity in mammalian lung. iv. Pulmonary lecithin synthesis in the human fetus and newborn and etiology of the respiratory distress syndrome. *Pediatr Res* 1972; **6**: 81-99.

60. Godfrey S. Respiratory and cardiovascular changes during asphyxia and resuscitation of foetal newborn rabbits. *Q J Exp Physiol Cogn Med Sci* 1968; **53**: 97-118.

61. Godfrey S. Blood gases during asphyxia and resuscitation of fetal and newborn rabbits. *Respir Physiol* 1968; **4**: 309-21.

62. Godfrey S, Bolton DPG, Cross KW. Respiratory stimulants in treatment of perinatal asphyxia. *Br Med J* 1970; **i**: 475-7.

63. Goldenberg RL, Huddleston JF, Nelson KG. Apgar scores and umbilical arterial pH in preterm infants. *Am J Obstet Gynecol* 1984; **149**: 651-4.

64. Halperin M. Heart massage in a newborn infant. *JAMA* 1957; **164**: 1996.

65. Hamer Hodges RJ, Tunstall ME, Knight RF, Wilson EJ. Endotracheal aspiration and oxygenation in resuscitation of the newborn. *Br J Anaesth* 1960; **32**: 9-15.

66. Hancock PJ, Peterson G. Finger intubation of the trachea in newborns. *Pediatrics* 1992; **89**: 325-6.

67. Handley DB, Handley D. A rocker for asphyxia neonatorum. *Br Med J* 1951; **ii**: 1282.

68. Hawdon JM, Ward Platt MP, Aynsley-Green A. Patterns of metabolic adaptation for preterm and term infants in the first neonatal week. *Arch Dis Child* 1992; **67**: 357-65.

69. Hawdon JM, Aynsley-Green A, Alberti KGMM, Ward Platt MP. The role of pancreatic insulin secretion in neonatal glucoregulation. 1. Healthy term and preterm infants. *Arch Dis Child* 1993; **68**: 274-9.

70. Hein HA. The use of sodium bicarbonate in neonatal resuscitation: help or harm? *Pediatrics* 1993; **91**: 496-7.

71. Hemingway A, Neil E. An experimental study of different methods of artificial respiration. *Br Med J* 1944; **i**: 833-6.

72. Henderson Y. The prevention and treatment of asphyxia in the newborn. *JAMA* 1928; **90**: 583-6.

73. Hey E, Hull D. Lung function at birth in babies developing respiratory distress. *J Obstet Gynaecol Br Commonw* 1971; **78**: 1137-46.

74. Hey E, Kelly J. Gaseous exchange during endotracheal ventilation for asphyxia at birth. *J Obstet Gynaecol Br Commonw* 1968; **75**: 414-24.

75. Hoseth E, Joergensen A, Ebbesen F, Moeller M. Blood glucose levels in a population of healthy, breast fed, term infants of appropriate size for gestational age. *Arch Dis Child Fetal Neonatal Ed* 2000; **83**: F117-19.

76. Hoskyns EW, Milner AD, Hopkin IE. A simple method of facemask resuscitation at birth. *Arch Dis Child* 1987; **62**: 376-8.

77. Hosono S, Inami I, Fujita H, *et al*. A role of end-tidal CO_2 monitoring for assessment of tracheal intubations in very low birth weight infants during neonatal resuscitation at birth. *J Perinat Med* 2009; **37**: 79–84.

78. Hughes SM, Blake BL, Woods SL, Lehmann CU. False-positive results on colorimetric carbon dioxide analysis in neonatal resuscitation: potential for serious patient harm. *J Perinatol* 2007; **27**: 800-1.

79. Hull D. Lung expansion and ventilation during resuscitation of asphyxiated newborn infants. *J Pediatr* 1969; **75**: 47-58.

80. Hutchison J, Kerr M, Williams K, Hopkinson W. Hyperbaric oxygen in the resuscitation of the newborn. *Lancet* 1963; **ii**: 1019-22.

81. Information & Statistics Division, Scottish Health Service. Hospital and Health Board Comparisons in Obstetrics 1988-90.1992; 57.

82. Ingimarsson J, Björklund LJ, Curstedt T. Incomplete protection by prophylactic surfactant against the adverse effects of large lung inflation in immature lambs at birth. *Intensive Care Med* 2004; **30**: 1446-53.

83. Jankov RP, Asztalos EV, Skidmore MB. Favourable neurological outcomes following delivery room cardiopulmonary resuscitation of infants < or = 750 g at birth. *J Paediatr Child Health* 2000; **36**: 19-22.

84. Jasani MS, Nadkarni VM, Finkelstein MS, *et al*. Effects of different techniques of endotracheal epinephrine administration in pediatric porcine hypoxic-hypercarbic cardiopulmonary arrest. *Crit Care Med* 1994; **22**: 1174–80.

85. Jobe AH, Kramer BW, Moss TJ *et al*. Decreased indicators of lung injury with continuous positive expiratory pressure in preterm lambs. *Pediatr Res* 2002; **52**: 387-92.

86. Johanson RB, Spencer SA, Rolfe P, *et al*. Effect of post-delivery care on neonatal body temperature. *Acta Paediatr* 1992; **81**: 859-63.

87. Johnson JWC, Richards DS, Wagaman RA. The case for routine umbilical blood acid-base studies at delivery. *Amer J Obstet Gynecol* 1990; **162**: 621-5.

88. Johnson KG, Babson SG. Resuscitation of the apneic premature infant. *Pediatrics* 1967; **40**: 99-100.

89. Johnston ED, Stenson BJ. Am I getting chest wall movement? *Arch Dis Child Fetal Neonatal Ed* 2010; 95: F391-2

90. Katz VL, Bowes WA Jr. Meconium aspiration syndrome: Reflections on a murky subject. *Am J Obstet Gynecol* 1992; **166**: 171-83.

91. Kempley ST, Moreiras JW, Petrone FL. Endotracheal tube length for neonatal intubation. *Resuscitation* 2008; **77**: 369-73.

92. Kendall GS, Kapetanakis A, Ratnavel N, *et al*. Passive cooling for initiation of therapeutic hypothermia in neonatal encephalopathy. *Arch Dis Child Fetal Neonatal Ed* 2010; **95**: F408-12.

93. Kent AL, Williams J. Increasing ambient operating theatre temperature and wrapping in polyethylene improves admission temperature in premature infants. *J Paediatr Child Health* 2008; **44**: 325-31.

94. Kleinman ME, Oh W, Stonestreet BS. Comparison of intravenous and endotracheal epinephrine during cardiopulmonary resuscitation in newborn piglets. *Crit Care Med* 1999; **27**: 2748-85.

95. Klinger G, Beyene J, Shah P, Perlman M. Do hyperoxaemia and hypercapnia add to the risk of brain injury after intrapartum asphyxia? *Arch Dis Child Fetal Neonatal Ed* 2005; **90**: 49-52.

96. Kluckow M, Evans N. Low systemic blood flow in the preterm infant. *Semin Neonatol* 2001; **6**: 75-84.

97. Knobel RB, Wimmer JE Jr, Holbert D. Heat loss prevention for preterm infants in the delivery room. *J Perinatol* 2005; **25**: 304-8.

98. Kouwenhoven WB, Jude JR, Knickerbocker GG. Closed-chest cardiac massage. *JAMA* 1960; **173**: 1064-7.

99. Kroll L, Twohey L, Daubeney PE, *et al*. Risk factors at delivery and the need for skilled resuscitation. *Eur J Obstet & Gynecol and Reprod Biol* 1994; **44**: 175-7.

100. Landon MB, Gabbe SG, Piana R, *et al*. Neonatal morbidity in pregnancy complicated by diabetes mellitus: predictive value of maternal glycemic profiles. *Amer J Obstet Gynecol* 1987; **156**: 1089-95.

101. Leahy FAN, Cates D, MacCallum M, Rigatto H. Effect of CO_2 and 100% O_2 on cerebral blood flow in preterm infants. *J Appl Physiol* 1980; **48**: 468-72.

102. Levene MI, Sands C, Grindulis H, Moore JR. Comparison of two methods of predicting outcome in perinatal asphyxia. *Lancet* 1986; **i**: 67-9.

103. Levene M. Cool treatment for asphyxia, but what's next? *Arch Dis Child Fetal Neonatal Ed* 2010; **95**: F154-7.

104. Lie KK, Grøholt EK, Eskild A. Association of cerebral palsy with Apgar score in low and normal birthweight infants: a population based cohort study. *Br Med J* 2010; **341**: c4990.

105. Lind J. Initiation of breathing in the newborn infant. *J Ir Med Assoc*. 1962; **50**: 88-93.

106. Lindemann R. Resuscitation of the newborn with endotracheal administration of epinephrine. *Acta Paed Scand* 1984; **73**: 210-2.

107. Linder N, Aranda JV, Tsur M, *et al*. Need for endotracheal intubation and suction in meconium stained neonates. *J Pediatr* 1988; **112**: 613-5.

108. Lindner W, Vofsbeck S,Hummler H, Pohldant F. Delivery room management of extremely low birth weight infants: spontaneous breathing or intubation? *Pediatrics* 1999; **103**: 961-7.

109. Macfarlane A, Mugford M. Birth counts; Statistics of pregnancy and childbirth. Chapter 12: 327-35. HMSO 2000.

110. Madar J, Richmond S, Hey E. Surfactant-deficient respiratory distress after elective delivery at 'term'. *Acta Paediatr* 1999; **88**: 1244-8.

111. Maskrey S. Neonatal resuscitation. *Clin Risk* 2008; **14**: 46-8.

112. McCall EM, Alderdice FA, Halliday HL, *et al*. Interventions to prevent hypothermia in preterm and/or low birthweight babies. Cochrane Database Syst Rev. 2008 Jan 23;(1):CD004210

113. Mead J. Paediatricians negligent in emergency: Antoniades v East Sussex Hospitals NHS Trust (High Court, 16/03/07 - Mackay J). *Clin Risk* 2008; **14**: 82-3.

114. Meltzer SJ. Simple devices for effective artificial respiration in emergencies. *JAMA* 1913; **60**: 1407-10.

115. Menegazzi JJ, Auble TE, Nicklas KA, *et al*. Two thumb versus two finger chest compression during CRP in a swine infant model of cardiac arrest. *Ann Emerg Med* 1993; **22**: 240-3.

116. Mercer JS, Vohr BR, McGrath MM, *et al*. Delayed cord clamping in very preterm infants reduces the incidence of intraventricular hemorrhage and late-onset sepsis - a randomized-controlled trial. *Pediatrics* 2006; **117**: 1235-42.

117. Mercer J, Erickson-Owens D, Skovgaard R. Cardiac asystole at birth: is hypovolemic shock the cause? *Med Hypotheses* 2009; **72**: 458-63.

118. Merritt TA, Farrell PM. Diminished pulmonary lecithin synthesis in acidosis: Experimental findings as related to the respiratory distress syndrome. *Pediatrics* 1976; **57**: 32-40.

119. Meyer A, Nadkarni V, Pollock A, *et al*. Evaluation of the Neonatal Resuscitation Program's recommended chest compression depth using computerized tomography imaging. *Resuscitation* 2010; **81**: 544-8.

120. Milner AD, Saunders RA. Pressure and volume changes in the first breath of human neonates. *Arch Dis Child* 1977; **52**: 918-24.

121. Modest VE, Butterworth JF 4th. Effect of pH and lidocaine on beta-adrenergic receptor binding: interaction during resuscitation. *Chest* 1995; **108**: 1373-9.

122. Moore WMO, Davis JA. Response of the newborn rabbit to acute anoxia and variations due to narcotic agents. *Br J Anaesth* 1966; **38**: 787-92.

123. Moreland TA, Brice JEM, Walker CHM, Parija AC. Naloxone pharmacokinetics in the newborn. *Br J Clin Pharmacol* 1979; **9**: 609-12.

124. Morley CJ, Davis PG, Doyle L, *et al*. Nasal CPAP or intubation for very preterm infants. *New Engl J Med* 2008; **358**: 700-8.

125. Moss AJ, Monset-Couchard M. Placental transfusion: early versus late clamping of the umbilical cord. *Pediatrics* 1967; **40**: 109-26.

126. Moya F, James LS, Bernard E, Hanks EC. Closed chest cardiac massage in the newborn. *Anaesthesiol* 1961; **22**: 644-5.

127. Nelson KB, Ellenberg JH. Apgar scores as predictors of chronic neurological disability. *Pediatrics* 1981; **68**: 36-44.

128. Oddie S, Wyllie J, Scally A. Use of self-inflating bags for neonatal resuscitation. *Resuscitation* 2005; **67**: 109-12.

129. O'Donnell AI, Gray PH, Rogers YM. Mortality and neurodevelopmental outcome for infants receiving adrenaline in neonatal resuscitation. *J Paediatr Child Health* 1988 **34**(6): 551-6.

130. O'Donnell CPF, Kamlin COF, Davis PG, Morley CJ. Obtaining pulse oximetry data in neonates: a randomised crossover study of sensor application techniques. *Arch Dis Child Fetal Neonatal Ed* 2005; **90**: F84-5.

131. O'Donnell CP, Kamlin CO, Davis PG, Morley CJ. Endotracheal intubation attempts during neonatal resuscitation: success rates, duration and adverse effects. *Pediatrics* 2006; **117**: e16-21

132. O'Donnell CPF, Kamlin COF, Davis PG, *et al*. Clinical assessment of infant colour at delivery. *Arch Dis Child Fetal Neonatal Ed* 2007; **92**: F465-7.

133. O'Donnell CPF, Stenson BJ. Respiratory strategies for preterm infants. *Semin Fetal Neonatal Med* 2008; **13**: 401-9.

134. Okumura A, Hayakawa F, Kato T *et al*. Hypocarbia in preterm infants with periventricular leukomalacia: the relation between hypocarbia and mechanical ventilation. *Pediatrics* 2001; **107**: 469-75.

135. Orlowski JP, Kanoti GA, Mehlman MJ. The ethics of using newly dead patients for teaching and practicing intubation techniques. *New Engl J Med* 1988; **319**: 439-41.

136. Owen CJ, Wyllie JP. Determination of heart rate in babies at birth. *Resuscitation* 2004; **60**: 213-7.

137. Palme C, Nyström B, Tunell R. An evaluation of the efficiency of facemasks in the resuscitation of newborn infants. *Lancet* 1985; **i**: 207-10.

138. Palme-Kilander C. Methods of resuscitation in low-Apgar-score in newborn infants -a national survey. *Acta Paediatr* 1992; **81**: 739-44.

139. Paterson SJ, Byrne PJ, Molesky MG, *et al*. Neonatal resuscitation using the laryngeal mask airway. *Anesthesiol* 1994; **80**: 1248-53.

140. Peltonen T. Placental transfusion - advantage and disadvantage. *Eur J Pediatr* 1981; **137**: 141-6.

141. Perlman JM, Risser R. Cardiopulmonary resuscitation in the delivery room. Associated clinical events. *Arch Pediatr Adolesc Med* 1995; **149**: 20-5.

142. Perlman JM, Wyllie J, Kattwinkel J, *et al*. Part 11: neonatal resuscitation: 2010 International consensus on cardiopulmonary resuscitation and emergency cardiovascular care science with treatment recommendations. *Circulation*. 2010; **122**(suppl 2): S516–38.

143. Phillips GW, Zideman DA. Relation of infant heart to sternum: its significance in cardiopulmonary resuscitation. *Lancet* 1986; **i**: 1024-5.

144. Plaat F. The team needs a leader. *Clinical Risk* 2008; **14**: 43-5.

145. Primhak RA, Herber SM, Whincup G, Milner RDG. Which deliveries require paediatricians in attendance? *Br Med J* 1984; **289**: 16-18.

146. Probyn ME, Hooper SB, Dargaville PA, *et al*. Positive end expiratory pressure during resuscitation of premature lambs rapidly improves blood gases without adversely affecting arterial pressure. *Pediatr Res* 2004; **56**: 198-204.

147. Rabe H, Reynolds G, Diaz-Rossello J. Early versus delayed umbilical cord clamping in preterm infants. *Cochrane Database of Systematic Reviews* 2004, Issue 4. Art No. CD003248.

148. Ramji S, Ahuja S, Thirupuram S, *et al*. Resuscitation of asphyxic newborn infants with room air or 100% oxygen. *Pediatr Res* 1993; **34**: 809-12.

149. Raymondos K, Panning B, Leuwer M *et al*. Absorption and hemodynamic effects of airway administration of adrenaline in patients with severe cardiac disease. *Ann Intern Med* 2000; **132**: 800-3.

150. Redding JS, Asuncion JS, Pearson JW. Effective routes of drug administration during cardiac arrest. *Anesth Analg (Clev)* 1967; **46**: 253-8.

151. Repetto JE, Donohue PK, Baker SF, *et al*. Use of capnography in the delivery room for assessment of endotracheal tube placement. *J Perinatol* 2001; **21**: 284–7.

152. Richmond S, Goldsmith JP. Refining the role of oxygen administration during delivery room resuscitation: What are the future goals? *Semin Fetal Neonatal Med* 2008; **13**: 368-74.

153. Richmond S, Wyllie J. European Resuscitation Council guidelines for resuscitation 2010. Section 7. Resuscitation of babies at birth. *Resuscitation* 2010; **81**: 1389-99.

154. Roberts WA, Maniscalco WM, Cohen AR, *et al*. The use of capnography for recognition of esophageal intubation in the neonatal intensive care unit. *Pediatr Pulmonol* 1995; **19**: 262–8.

155. Robertson CMT, Finer NN, Grace MGA. School performance in survivors of neonatal encephalopathy associated with birth asphyxia at term. *J Pediatr* 1989; **114**: 753-60.

156. Royal College of Midwives. Home birth handbook volume 1: promoting home birth. RCM London 2002.

157. Royal College of Midwives. Home birth handbook volume 2: practising home birth. RCM London 2003.

158. RCOG Scientific Advisory Committee. Clamping of the umbilical cord and placental transfusion. Royal College of Obstetricians and Gynaecologists Opinion Paper 14, 2009.

159. Rudikoff MT, Maughan WL, Effron M, *et al*. Mechanisms of blood flow during cardiopulmonary resuscitation. *Circulation* 1980; **61**: 345-52.

160. Safar P, Escarraga LA, Elam JO. A comparison of the mouth-to-mouth and mouth-to-airway methods of artificial respiration with chest-pressure arm-lift methods. *N Engl J Med* 1958; **258**: 671-7.

161. Sarnat HB, Sarnat MS. Neonatal encephalopathy following fetal distress: a clinical and electroencephalographic study. *Arch Neurol* 1976; **33**: 696-705.

162. Saugstad OD, Rootwelt T, Aalen O. Resuscitation of asphyxiated newborn infants with room air or oxygen: an international controlled trial: the Resair 2 study. *Pediatrics* 1998; **102**: e1.

163. Schmölzer GM, Kamlin COF, Dawson JA. *et al*. Respiratory monitoring of neonatal resuscitation. *Arch Dis Child Fetal Neonatal Ed* 2010; **95**: F295-303.

164. Schmölzer GM, Kamlin COF, O'Donnell CPF *et al*. Assessment of tidal volume and gas leak during mask inflation of preterm infants in the delivery room. *Arch Dis Child Fetal Neonatal Ed* 2010; doi: 10.1136/adc.2009.174003.

165. Shankaran S (ed). Perinatal asphyxia. *Clin Perinatol* 1993; **20**: 287-505.

166. Sims DG, Heal CA, Bartle SM. The use of adrenaline and atropine in neonatal resuscitation. *Arch Dis Child* 1994; **70**: F3-10.

167. Skellet S, Mayer A, Durward A, *et al*. Chasing the base deficit: hyperchloraemic acidosis following 0·9% saline fluid resuscitation. *Arch Dis Child* 2000; **83**: 514-6.

168. Spevak MR, Kleinman PK, Belanger PL, *et al*. Cardiopulmonary resuscitation and rib fractures in infants; a postmortem radiologic-pathologic study. *JAMA* 1994; **272**: 617-8.

169. Stanley FJ, Alberman ED. Infants of very low birthweight. 1. Factors affecting survival. *Dev Med Child Neurol* 1978; **20**: 300-12.

170. Steiner H, Neligan GA. Perinatal cardiac arrest: quality of the survivors. *Arch Dis Child* 1975; **50**: 696-702.

171. Stenson B. Resuscitation of extremely preterm infants: The influence of positive pressure, surfactant replacement and supplemental oxygen on outcome. Hansen TN, McIntosh N (eds) Current Topics in Neonatology No 4. WB Saunders, London, 2000.

172. Stephens RH, Benjamin AR, Walters DV. Volume and protein concentration of epithelial lining liquid in perfused in situ postnatal sheep lungs. *Am J Physiol* 1996; **80**: 1911-20.

173. Stephenson JM, Du JN, Oliver TK. The effect of cooling on blood gas tensions in newborn infants. *J Pediatr* 1970; **76**: 848-51.

174. Stevens SS. On the theory of scales of measurement. *Science* 1946; **103**: 677-80.

175. Strang LB. Fetal lung liquid: secretion and reabsorption. *Physiological Reviews* 1991; **71**: 991-1016.

176. Sutherland JM, Epple HH. Cardiac massage of stillborn infants. *Obstet Gynecol* 1961; **18**: 182-6.

177. Sykes G, Molloy P, Johnson P, *et al*. Do Apgar scores indicate asphyxia? *Lancet* 1982; **i**: 494-6.

178. Tan A, Schulze A, O'Donnell CPF, Davis PG. Air versus oxygen for resuscitation of infants at birth (Cochrane Review). In: The Cochrane Library, Issue 3, 2004. Chichester, UK: John Wiley & Sons, Ltd.

179. te Pas AB, Walther FJ. A randomized, controlled trial of delivery-room respiratory management in very preterm infants. *Pediatrics* 2007; **120**: 322-9.

180. Thaler MM, Stobie GHC. An improved technique of external cardiac compression in infants and young children. *New Eng J Med* 1963; **269**: 606-10.

181. The OSIRIS collaborative group. Early versus delayed neonatal administration of a synthetic surfactant - the judgement of OSIRIS. *Lancet* 1992; **340**; 1363-9.

182. Thiebault DW, Hall FK, Sheehan MB, Hall RT. Postasphyxial lung disease in newborn infants with severe perinatal acidosis. *Am J Obstet Gynecol* 1984; **150**: 393-9.

183. Thió M, Bhatia R, Dawson JA *et al*. Oxygen delivery using neonatal self-inflating bags without a reservoir. *Arch Dis Child Fetal Neonatal Ed* 2010; **95**: F315-9.

184. Tin W, Wariyar U, Hey E. Changing prognosis for babies of less than 28 weeks gestation in the north of England between 1983 and 1994. *Br Med J* 1997; **314**: 107-11.

185. Todres ID, Rogers MC. Methods of external cardiac massage in the newborn infant. *J Pediatr* 1975; **86**: 781-2.

186. Tolosa JN, Dong-Hyuk P, Eve DJ *et al*. Mankind's first natural stem cell transplant. *J. Cell. Mol. Med.* 2010; **14**: 488-95.

187. Tonkin SL, Davis SL, Gunn TR. Nasal route for infant resuscitation by mothers. *Lancet* 1995; **345**: 1353-4.

188. Tracy M, Downe L, Holberton J. How safe is intermittent positive pressure ventilation in preterm babies ventilated from delivery to newborn intensive care unit. *Arch Dis Child Fetal Neonatal Ed* 2004; **89**: F84-7.

189. Tracy MB, Klimek J, Coughtrey H, *et al*. Mask leak in one-person mask ventilation compared to two-person in a newborn infant manikin study. *Arch Dis Child Fetal Neonatal Ed* 2010; doi: 10.1136/adc.2009.169847

190. Tunstall ME, Hodges RJH. A sterile disposable neonatal tracheal tube. *Lancet* 1961; **i**: 146.

191. UKCC Standards for Records and Record Keeping. London 1993, UKCC.

192. Upton CJ, Milner AD. Endotracheal resuscitation of neonates using a rebreathing bag. *Arch Dis Child* 1991; **66**: 39-42.

193. Vain NE, Szyld EG, Prudent LM, *et al*. Oropharyngeal and nasopharyngeal suctioning of meconium-stained neonates before delivery of their shoulders: multicentre, randomised controlled trial. *Lancet* 2004; **364**: 597-602.

194. Vanhaesebrouck P, Vanneste K, de Praeter C, *et al*. Tight nuchal cord and neonatal hypovolaemic shock. *Arch Dis Child* 1987; **62**: 1276-7.

195. Verder H, Albertsen P, Ebbesen F. *et al*. Nasal continuous positive airway pressure and early surfactant therapy for respiratory distress syndrome in newborns of less than 30 weeks gestation. *Pediatrics* 1999; **103**: e24.

196. Vohra S, Roberts RS, Zhang B, *et al*. Heat Loss Prevention (HeLP) in the delivery room: A randomized controlled trial of polyethylene occlusive skin wrapping in very preterm infants. *J Pediatr* 2004; **145**: 750-3.

197. Vyas H, Milner AD, Hopkin IE, Boon AW. Physiologic responses to prolonged and slow rise inflation in the resuscitation of the asphyxiated newborn infant. *J Pediatr* 1981; **99**: 635-9.

198. Walters DW, Olver RE. The role of catecholamines in lung liquid absorption at birth. *Pediatr Res* 1978; **12**: 239-42.

199. Westgate J, Garibaldi JM, Greene KR. Umbilical cord blood gas analysis at delivery; a time for quality data. *Br J Obstet Gynaecol* 1994; **101**: 1054-63.

200. Westin B, Miller J, Nyberg R, Wedenberg E. Neonatal asphyxia pallida treated with hypoperfusion and transfusion of oxygenated blood. *Surgery* 1959; **45**: 868-79.

201. Whyte SD, Sinha AK, Wyllie JP. Neonatal resuscitation – a practical assessment. *Resuscitation* 1999; **40**: 21-5.

202. Wilkinson AR (chairman) BPA working party. Neonatal resuscitation. British Paediatric Association, London 1993.

203. Wilkinson AR, Ahluwalia J, Cole A, *et al*. Management of babies born extremely preterm at less than 26 weeks of gestation: a framework for clinical practice at the time of birth. *Arch Dis Child Fetal Neonatal Ed* 2009; **94**: F2-5.

204. Wiswell TE, Gannon CM, Jacob J, *et al*. Delivery room management of the apparently vigorous meconium-stained neonate: results of the multicenter international collaborative trial. *Pediatrics* 2000; **105**: 1-7.

205. Wood NS, Marlow N, Costeloe K, *et al*. Neurologic and developmental disability after extremely preterm birth. *N Engl J Med* 2000; **343**: 374-84.

206. Woody NC, Woody HB. Direct digital intratracheal intubation for neonatal resuscitation. *J Pediatr* 1968; **73**: 903-5.

207. World Health Organisation. WHO recommendations for the prevention of postpartum haemorrhage. Making pregnancy safer. 2007

208. Wyckoff MH, Perlman JM, Laptook AR. Use of volume expansion during delivery room resuscitation in near-term and term infants. *Pediatrics* 2005; **115**: 950-5.

209. Wyllie J, Perlman J, Kattwinkel J *et al*. 2010 International consensus on cardiopulmonary resuscitation and emergency cardiovascular care science with treatment recommendations: Neonatal resuscitation. *Resuscitation* 2010; **81S**: e260-87.

210. Yao AC, Hirvensalo M, Lind J. Placental transfusion-rate and uterine contraction. *Lancet* 1968; **i**: 380-3

211. Yao AC, Lind J. Effect of gravity on placental transfusion. *Lancet* 1969; **ii**: 505-8.

NLS

Index

WITHDRAWN